LEARNING SURGICAL TECHNIQUE: BASIC SKILLS

A Practical Guide

By

ALEXANDR I. LEMESCHEWSKIJ

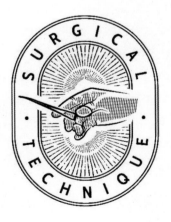

The author would like to express his thanks to Sviatlana A. Klimuk MD and to Ben Hooson PhD for their assistance in the translation and preparation of the English version of Learning Surgical Technique: Basic Skills.

This practical guide for the development of the surgeon's hands offers a detailed introduction to basis surgery, together with a series of exercises. It can be used to accompany the early stages of a training in surgery, for reference and practice in later stages, and will also be useful to surgeons with practical experience who want to systematize their knowledge and improve their skills. Starting from initial exercises to develop finger and hand dexterity, the book moves on to detailed explanations of loops, knots and sutures, instructions in the handling of surgical instruments, and an overview of suture materials. The explanations are designed to be simple and clear, and each explanation is accompanied by a diagram. The exercises will foster all of the key hand skills that are essential for work in the operating theatre: accuracy, coordination, confidence, plasticity of movement, strength, endurance, correct hold of surgical instruments, etc. Treated as a course of study with adequate time devoted to the exercises, the book can be worked through in three to four months, assuming 20 to 30 minutes of study and practice each day.

DEDICATION

To my grandmother, Anna, in gratitude for her constant love, faith and assistance.
To my family for their support and understanding.
To my teachers for their inspiration, wisdom and patience.
To my students for their attention and hope for the future.
To my patients for their trust and respect.

Becoming a surgeon is a difficult but marvelous road to travel, and a source of inner pride for whoever has travelled it.

INTRODUCTION

This book is about the surgeon's hands. Its aim is to develop hand skills and dexterity in someone who has decide to devote their life to surgery. The exercises described in the book will foster a number of key hand skills that are essential for the work in the operating theatre: accuracy, coordination, confidence, plasticity of movement, strength, endurance, correct hold of surgical instruments, etc.

Completion of the course will prepare the student for the next stages of practical training. Surgeons who already have practical experience will find the book useful for systematizing their knowledge and for improving the skills, which they already have. Main benefits of the descriptions and practical exercises, contained in the book, are as follows:

- You will unlock the potential of your hands, improving your performance as a surgeon.
- You will learn (by completing the first half of the book) the theory and practice of the correct creation of loops and knots, which is perhaps the most vital skill for a surgeon.
- Subtleties and "knacks" of basic surgery are revealed, and the most common errors are explained.
- As you work through the book you will experience gradual increase of hand dexterity and, after completion of the whole training course, you will notice the benefit for your work in the operating theatre.
- Working through the book will lay firm foundations for quick learning of new surgery skills.
- Your confidence in your own hands will be much increased.

The Author of the book has 23 years' experience as a surgeon, including 16 years as a teacher of surgery at a Medical University. The skills that are explained and the way they are explained reflect what the author has learnt about the best and most fruitful ways of teaching surgery. The effectiveness of the training path followed in the book has been proven by learning outcomes over many years.

The focus of the book is practical, descriptions are supported by pictures for ease of understanding, and the importance of each hand skill in surgical practice is explained. Despite the author's best efforts, it is always possible that some points in the book are not fully clear and that implementation by the student will differ from what the Autor intended.
A video course will create in order to address this and to ensure that students acquire best-possible techniques and habits from the outset.

Completion of the studies and exercises set out in the book should take about three to four months (approximately one week for each topic), assuming that you will devote 20 to 30 minutes to them each day. Each new skill should be practiced for about three weeks.

TABLE OF CONTENTS

TOPIC 11

TOPIC 12

TOPIC 13

TOPIC 1.

FIRST EXERCISES. TRAINING APPARATUS. TRAINING PLAN

Training with matches

Hand training with matches may seem too elementary for the aspiring surgeon, but aching muscles after the first few exercises will prove the opposite. The following match exercises should be mastered until they become second nature.

A box of matches is all that one needs to start.

Do the exercises with the right hand and then the left hand. When proficiency attained, practice the exercises simultaneously with both hands.

In all of the exercises the matches are gripped, one-by-one and end-to-end, between the flat sides of the thumb (1) and of each finger (2-5): 1–2, 1–3, 1–4, 1–5. Fig. 1.1 shows the four possible grips. The purpose of the exercises is to increase the grip strength of thumbs and fingers.

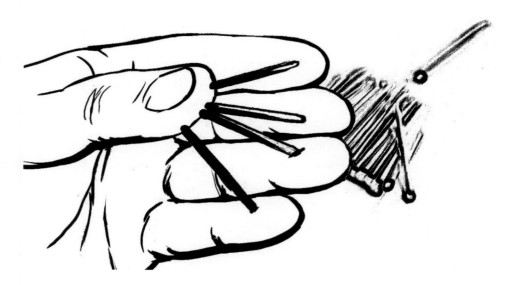

Fig. 1.1. Match grips for the exercises

1

Match-picking exercise

Try to do this exercise quickly. Shake the matches out of the box and put them back again one by one, grabbing them at the two ends between fingers 1–2, 1–3, 1–4, 1–5 in turn (Figs. 1.2–1.5).

Task. Practice match picking with the fingers of the right and left hands.

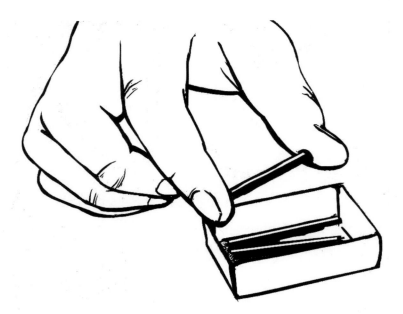

Fig. 1.2. Match picking with fingers 1–2

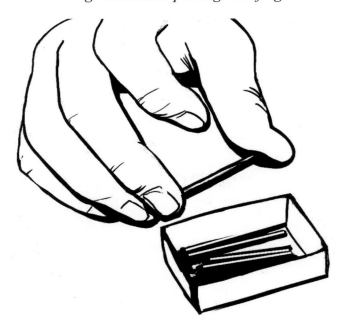

Fig. 1.3. Match picking with fingers 1–3

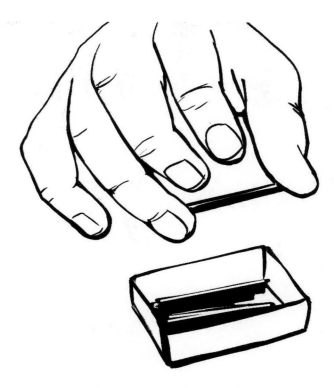

Fig. 1.4. Match picking with fingers 1–4

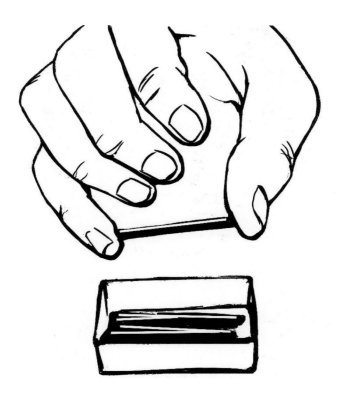

Fig. 1.5. Match picking with fingers 1–5

Well-building exercise

In this exercise the student builds a "well" out of matches, grabbing the matches between alternate fingers, as in the previous exercise, and placing them on top of each other as shown (Figs. 1.6–1.7).

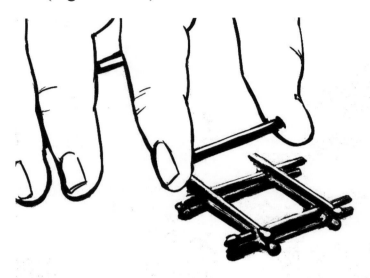

Fig. 1.6. Match picking with fingers 1–2 to build a well

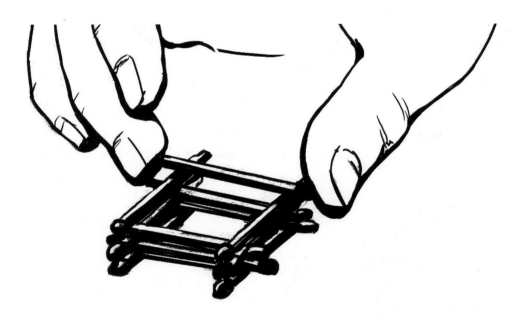

Fig. 1.7. Match picking with fingers 1–3 to build a well

When doing the exercises, notice that the matches fall if they are not held firmly enough, but they stick to the finger (especially the head of the match) if they are held too firmly. Work to avoid both.

Berry-picking exercise

The challenge here is to gather four matches in the palm of the collecting hand before putting them in the box. Again, the matches are grabbed at the two ends, one by one, alternating between different pairs of fingers and different hands (Fig. 1.8).

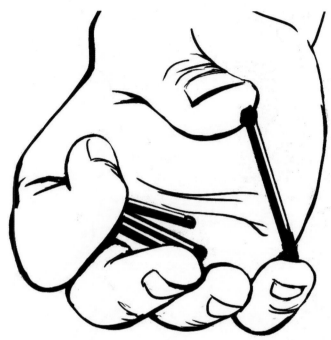

Fig. 1.8. Gripping the fourth match with fingers 1–5 in the berry-picking exercise (finger–2 holds down three previously collected matches)

Task. Master the match exercises, working with both hands at the same time.

SELF-ASSESSMENT

The student can judge when he/she has mastered the exercises based on simple criteria:
- the exercise is performed more confidently and quickly;
- the right and left hands perform the exercise equally well (it can help to hold a "competition" between right and left hands, and the most satisfactory result is that the dominant hand comes off worse);
- movements become automatic.

Different people achieve facility differently, but it always takes time. On average, you will need about three weeks to achieve mastery, followed by regular repetition to retain it.

TERMINOLOGY

Every discipline has its own specialized terminology, generated by years of research and practice. The present book uses some terms that may not be immediately understandable, even for a reader with some knowledge of surgery (for instance, in describing how to tie knots correctly). Explanations provided where necessary.

Preparing a training apparatus

The student will require his/her own simple set of instruments and other items in order to carry out the tasks described below.

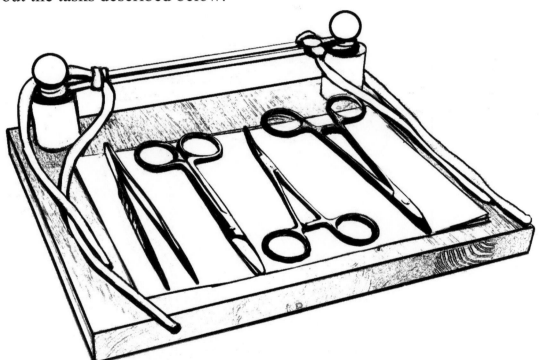

Fig. 1.9. A basic training apparatus and instruments

It is a good idea to have a few basic instruments and an apparatus ready and waiting before you embark on the tasks below. A suitable set, with tried and tested ergonomics, is shown in Fig. 1.9. It includes instruments, a surface with two posts and double soft tube to practice suture techniques, thread and other components. It has the advantages of being compact and including everything you will need to learn core techniques.
Task. Prepare the training apparatus and a place to train.

6

Selection of a surgical clamp for training

You will need a medium-sized surgical clamp (hemostatic clamp, Billroth clamp), which must be light, well-balanced and ergonomic, i.e., right for your hand.

It is a good idea to use brand-new instruments for the training tasks described below, because this will teach the student how much easier it is to work with a new instrument and when it is time to replace one that is no longer fit for use.

The clamp must be neither too long or too short, but about the same length as the hand. If the clamp is not brand new, check that its condition is adequate: the shanks should open easily and thick thread should be firmly held when the ratchet is moved by two clicks. "Pensioned off" instruments, which are still adequate for student use, sometimes may be obtained from operating theatres.

Note that the ratchet should be located on the inner surface of the clamp rings (Fig. 1.10). Any other positioning of the ratchet is not suitable for the most common tasks. An inappropriately designed instrument will make it harder to carry out the exercises below.

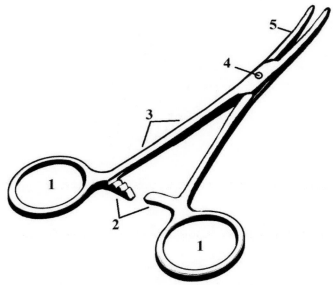

Fig. 1.10. Parts of a surgical clamp: 1 – rings; 2 – ratchet; 3– shank; 4 – joint; 5 – jaws and tip

Many surgical instruments share the basic design of the clamp. Make sure you are familiar with its parts (Fig. 1.10), since they will often be referred to in description of the exercises below.

First exercises with a surgical clamp

The purpose of the first exercises with the clamp is to accustom fingers and hands to the closing and opening mechanism. It may take some time to achieve ease of hand movement.

Learn how to close and open the clamp with fingers 1–4 (one and four) of both right and left hands in the rings (Fig. 1.11). If the tip of the clamp is curved, the curve should always be directed inwards (towards an imaginary perpendicular line midway between the hands).

When closing and opening the clamp, finger–2 is held by the joint of the clamp, and finger–3 helps the finger–4 to control the lower shank. Movement should be smooth, without jerks.

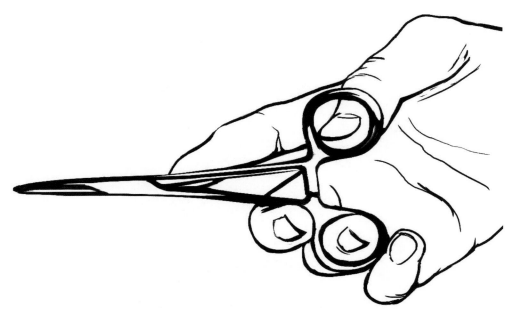

Fig. 1.11. Holding the surgical clamp with fingers–1–4 of the right hand. Concave surface of the clamp faces the midline.

Important to note: A surgeon's basic kit contains a minimum set of instruments. A surgical hemostatic clamp has pride of place in the set, since it can be used both for its principal purpose (temporary sealing of blood vessels) and also for the extraction of foreign bodies (for example, from the external auditory canal), removal of a tick, examination of a wound, stitching, etc.

Next, try closing and opening the clamp with fingers–1–3 of each hand in the rings (Fig. 1.12).

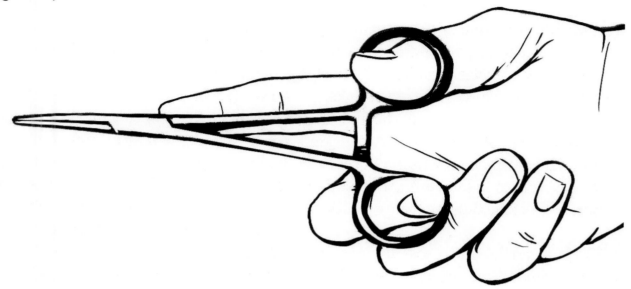

Fig. 1.12. Holding the clamp with fingers–1–3 of the right hand

Task. Practice closing and opening the clamp with fingers–1–4 and 1–3 of each hand.

Using a surgical clamp in match exercises

Use the clamp to grab matches without closing the ratchet and the match-picking and well-building exercises described above (Figs 1.13, 1.14).

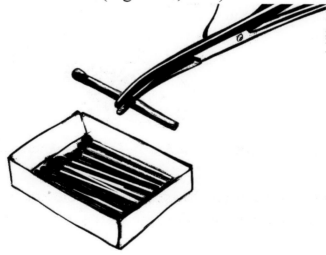

Fig. 1.13. Match-picking exercise using the surgical clamp

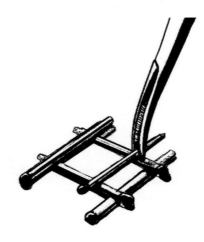

Fig. 1.14. Well-building exercise using the surgical clamp

Task. Master the match-picking and well-building exercises with right and left hands using the surgical clamp.

Gripping threads

There are several ways of gripping threads using the fingers: frontal grip, wrapped around the finger, and grip between the sides of fingers.

The following exercises develop the various thread grips.

The exercise uses a lace rather than an actual thread. The lace should be about 60 cm long, soft, elastic and not too thick (thick and hard lace is difficult to manipulate).

Use a lace of two different colors, for example 30 cm white and 30 cm black, since this makes it easier to see how knots are constructed (this will be discussed in detail below).

Main thread grips:

➢ **Frontal grip:**
  • fingers 1–2 (Fig. 1.15);
  • fingers 1–3 (Fig. 1.16).
➢ **Grip with sides of fingers:**
  • fingers 2–3 (Fig. 1.17).
➢ **Frontal grip:**
  • fingers 3–4–5 (Fig. 1.18);
  • fingers 4–5 (Fig. 1.19).

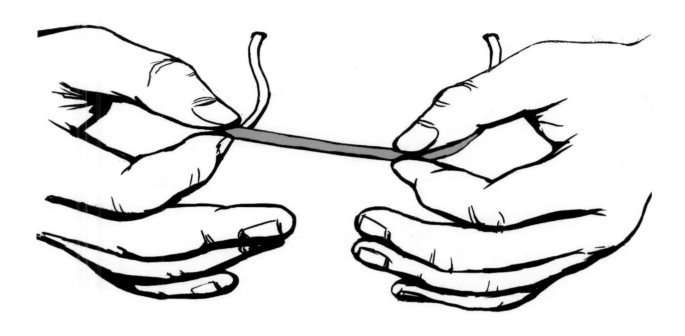

Fig. 1.15. Frontal grip with fingers 1–2

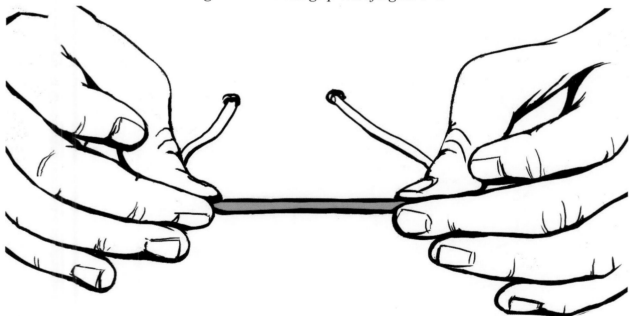

Fig. 1.16. Frontal grip with fingers 1–3

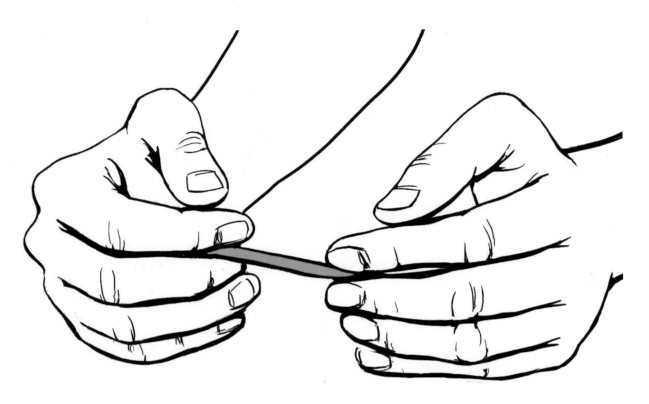

Fig. 1.17. Grip with sides of fingers 2–3

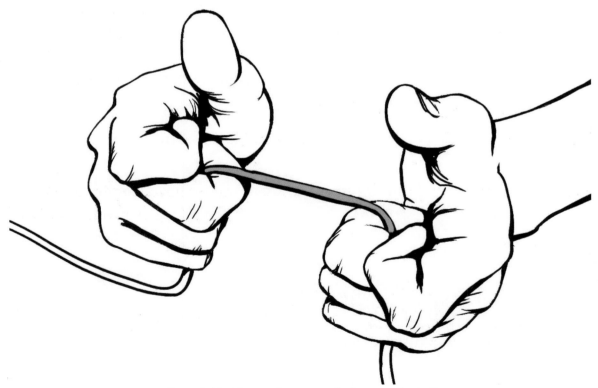

Fig. 1.18. Frontal grip with fingers 3–4–5

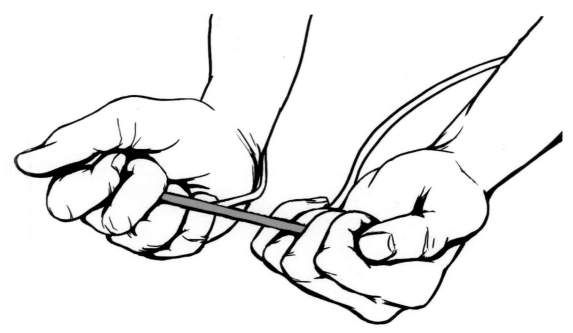

Fig. 1.19. Frontal grip with fingers 4–5

Practise these grips one after another with both hands in the order in which they are described. First, practise the grip with front of fingers 1–2, then with front of fingers 1–3, then grip the lace with sides of fingers 2–3, followed by the grip with fingers 3–4–5, and finally with fingers 4–5. Repeat the exercises over and again from the start.

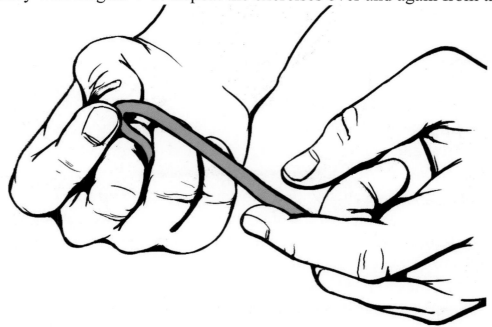

Fig. 1.20. Uncoordinated transition from grip with front of fingers 4–5 to grip with front of fingers 1–2

13

The point of the sequence and repetition is to develop smooth transition from one thread grip to another, with good coordination between the hands. Try to avoid loss of coordination (as in the example of Fig. 1.20).

Tasks. 1. Practise the grips in the sequence described.

2. Practise the grips in different sequences.

Training recommendations

Use of threads or laces in the exercises. Movement of threads in the wrong direction when tying a knot (twisting or crossing the threads) weakens the strength of the knot, with a risk that it will come undone after the operation.

Use of thin thread makes it hard to tell whether a knot has been tied correctly, so it is highly recommended to use a lace, and not thread, when learning how to form loops and knots. The words "thread" and "lace" are interchangeable in what follows, but it should always be understood that a lace is to be used.

When doing the exercises, pay attention to the movement of your fingers. You will see and feel the structure of the knots more easily as you practise.

Practice with right and left hands. One hand usually leads when making a loop. For purposes of the exercises below it is assumed that, when the movements are being learnt for the first time, the leading hand is the right hand. All of the explanations and illustrations make that assumption. People who are left–handed can decide for themselves whether to reverse this. It is worth noting that, in practice, the left hand needs to be more dexterous than the right, since it has to make loops more often than the right hand. This is explained further on.

Ways of making loops. Making loops by passing threads from one hand to the other is inefficient. In addition, a surgeon who gets used to doing this may occasionally omit to do it, in which case the threads are crossed and the loop or the whole knot may come undone. Sticky gloves (smeared with wound contents), thin thread and shortage of time are additional arguments against transferring the thread between hands.

Work speed. Rapid work by the surgeon's hands only impresses if the patient makes a rapid recovery. Do not make fast work an aim in itself when carrying out the exercises. Haste leads to bad habits, which are hard to get rid of.

Stance of the surgeon relative to the wound. Ideally, the edges of the wound should be parallel to a straight line between the surgeon's elbows. When doing the exercises, the training apparatus should always be placed accordingly (Fig. 1.21). In this position the end of the thread under the stretched tubes of the training apparatus is referred to as the start of the thread, and the other end is called the end of the thread.

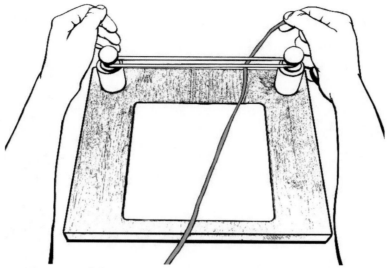

Fig. 1.21. Correct positioning of the training apparatus. The end of the thread is in the right hand

TEST QUESTIONS AND TASKS

1.1. Which match exercises can be carried out simultaneously with both hands?

1.2. Name the parts of a surgical clamp.

1.3. What is wrong with the handgrip on the clamp shown in Fig. 1.22?

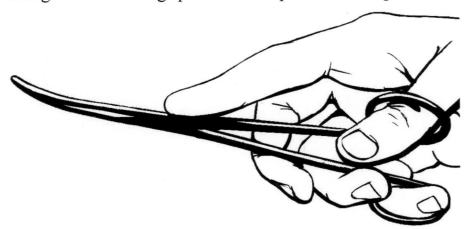

Fig. 1.22. Incorrect clamp grip

1.4. Describe the thread grip shown in Fig.1.23.

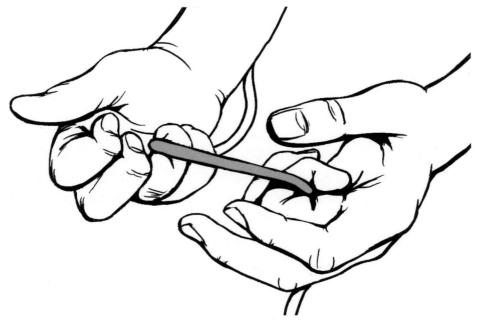

Fig. 1.23. Thread grip

1.5. What is the ideal length of the lace used for training? Is this the length of the lace, which you are using?

1.6. Explain the best stance of the student relative to the training apparatus.

1.7. Why is it not recommended to make loops and knots by passing threads from hand to hand?

TOPIC 2.

LOOPS AND KNOTS

The concept of loop and knot

Surgical suture is the connection of human tissues using thread. The thread is anchored in the tissue by the making of knots (Fig. 2.1). Knots consist of loops. Loops can be right or left, simple or complex.

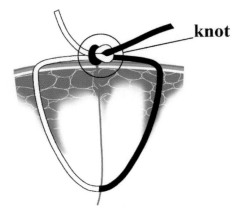

Fig. 2.1. Connection of tissue by surgical suture

Knots consist of loops, which are the main structural elements of any knot. A loop is the crossing of two ends of a thread to make a circle. The tightening of loops forms a knot (Fig. 2.2).

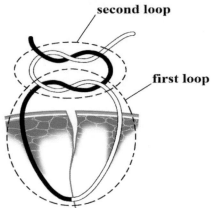

Fig. 2.2. Structure of a knot

18

A single tightened loop is called a "simple knot" (Fig. 2.3).

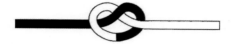

Fig. 2.3. Formation of a simple knot

Task. Make a knot on the training apparatus (see Fig. 2.2). Identify the first and second loops.

Right and left loops

If the start of the thread comes out of the loop to the right, the loop is a right loop (Fig. 2.4). If the start of the thread comes out of the loop to the left, the loop is a left loop (Fig. 2.5).

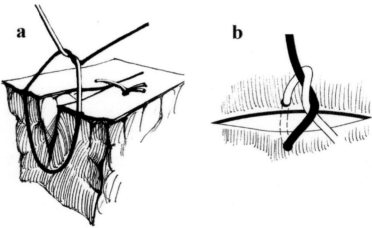

Fig. 2.4. Making a right loop (a, b)

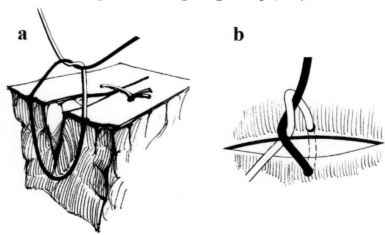

Fig. 2.5. Making a left loop (a, b)

Tasks. 1. Take two laces and make right and left loops on the training apparatus.
2. Make sure that the loops are evenly shaped.
After making a right or left loop, turn the training apparatus 180 degrees. Note that the form of the loop is the same, whichever side you look at it from: it is still a left or right loop (you can convince yourself of this more simply by turning Fig. 2. by 180 degrees).

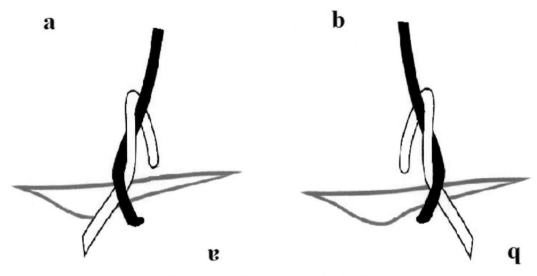

Fig. 2.6. Left (a) and right (b) loops

By carrying out the last exercise, you will have realized that there are only two kinds of simple loop – right and left. This seems too obvious to deserve saying, but it has an important consequence: **there are many ways of making loops, but whichever way you do it, you always obtain either a right or a left loop.**

20

Rule of loop alternation

When you make a knot, the loops must always alternate (Fig. 2.7):

    right – left – right – left, etc.

or

    left – right – left – right, etc.

In whatever way you form loops to make a knot, you must always alternate the loops (right – left) and tighten them properly.

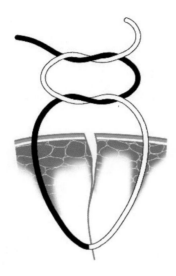

Fig. 2.7. Right loop followed by left loop

Task. What are the directions of the loops in Fig. 2.8? Do they alternate or not?

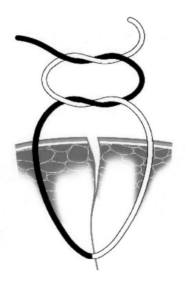

Fig. 2.8. A knot with two loops

Complex loops

Complex loops have several weaves (Figs. 2.9, 2.10).

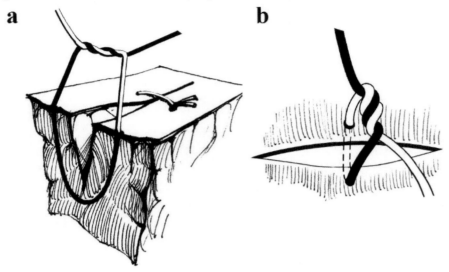

Fig. 2.9. Making a complex double-right loop (a, b)

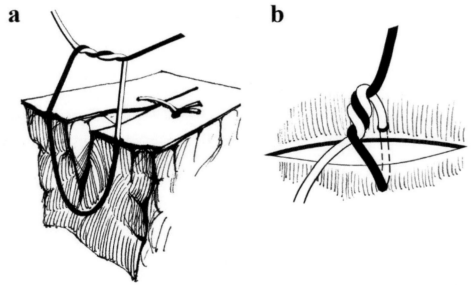

Fig. 2.10. Making a complex double-left loop (a, b)

Task. Make right and left loops with two weaves.
(This task is only intended to show that one loop can include several thread weaves. The actual technique of making complex loops will be discussed further on).

Coding of loops and knots

In 1983, L. Meiss proposed a code for describing knots, where a right loop was denoted by "+", a left loop by "−", and the number of weaves in the loop were described by a digit.

Examples of knots

Crossed knot, +1+1 or −1−1 (Fig. 2.11). The crossed knot is not recommended for use in surgery as the loops are one–directional, making the knot insecure.

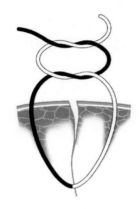

Fig. 2.11. Crossed knot +1+1

The most commonly used knots in surgery are the square, surgeon's and academic knots.

The structure of the square knot is +1−1 or −1+1 (Fig. 2.12). It can be continued to make a double square knot (+1−1+1 or −1+1−1) and a triple square knot (+1−1+1−1 or −1+1−1+1).

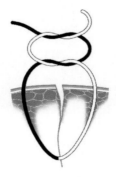

Fig. 2.12. Square knot, +1−1

The structure of the surgeon's knot is +2–1 or –2+1 (Fig. 2.13). It can be continued to make a double surgeon's knot (+2–1+1 or –2+1–1) and a triple surgeon's knot (+2–1+1–1 or –2+1–1+1).

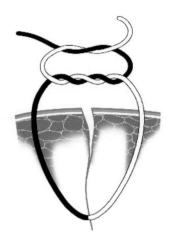

Fig. 2.13. Surgeon's knot, +2–1

The structure of the academic knot is +2–2 or –2+2 (Fig. 2.14). It can be continued to make a double academic knot (+2–2+2 or –2+2–2). Variants for continuation of the academic knot are +2–2+1 or –2+2–1, 2–2+1–1, and +2–2+1–1 or –2+2–1+1.

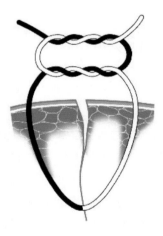

Fig. 2.14. Academic knot, +2–2

If the square, surgeon's and academic knots are strengthened with additional loops, these loops must also alternate in direction. The decision how may loops be use in a knot depends on many factors and will be discussed later.

Tasks. 1. Use the knot code to describe the square, surgeon's and academic knots.
2. State the rule of loop alternation.

Thread hold and loop direction

The following relationships between thread hold and loop direction applies to all the ways of making loops that are described below (Fig. 2.15): **if the end of the thread is held by the right hand, a right loop is made; if the end of the thread is held by the left hand, a left loop is made.**
So, the direction of the loop is the same as the hand (right or left), which holds the end of the thread.

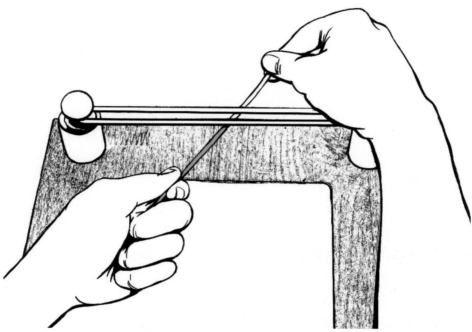

Fig. 2.15. The end of the thread is in the right hand, a right loop is made

In what follows we will use the phrases, "way of making a loop for the end of the thread" and "way of making a loop for the start of the thread" to indicate which hand leads or dominates in making a loop and which hand holds the start or end of the thread.

Rule of thread movement

After each loop, the ends of the thread are reversed: the end becomes the start and the start becomes the end (Fig. 2.16). Correct movement of the threads is the key to proper formation of the knot. Always keep this in mind.

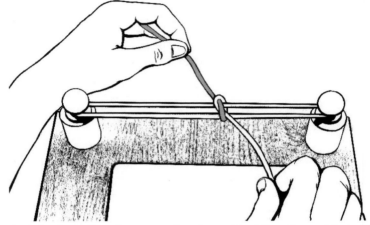

Fig. 2.16. A right loop has been made; the end of the thread is in the left hand

When the hands are moving correctly, making of the knot resembles the operation of a two-cylinder engine (Fig. 2.17). This is because the thread is not shifted from hand to hand, and hands and threads move only forwards or backwards. Each thread is alternately end and start, changing its position after each loop, but staying in the same hand throughout.

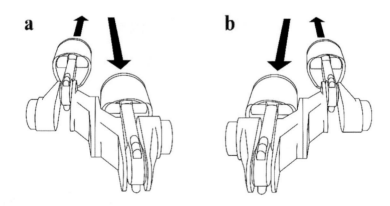

Fig. 2.17. Hand movement in loop making resembles the operation of a two-cylinder engine (a, b)

Always remember: when the start of the thread emerges from a loop, it becomes the end, and the end becomes the start; however, the threads are not shifted from hand to hand, but each remains in the same hand.

Tasks. 1. State the rule of thread movement. 2. State the rule for the relationship between thread hold and loop direction.

Hand pronation and supination

The terms "pronation" and "supination" (Fig. 2.18) will be used in the description of loop–making techniques.

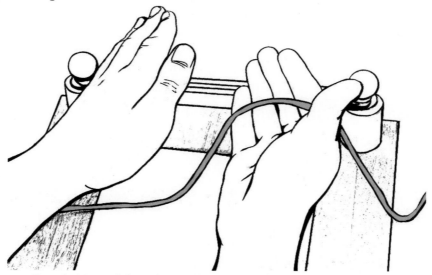

Fig. 2.18. Left hand in pronation, right hand in supination

Pronation is the revolution of the hand to a palm-down position.
Supination is the revolution of the hand to a palm-up position.

TEST QUESTIONS AND TASKS

2.1. A knot is made of loops. Give the definition of a loop.

2.2. In Fig. 2.19 what is the name of the part of the knot, which is circled by a broken line. What is the code of this knot using the Meiss system?

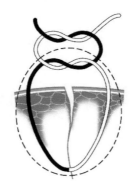

Fig. 2.19. Structure of a knot

2.3. Name the loop in Fig. 2.20, and give its Meiss code.

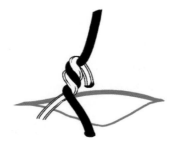

Fig. 2.20. A loop

2.4. Which is the left loop and which is the right loop as shown in Fig. 2.21?

a   **b**

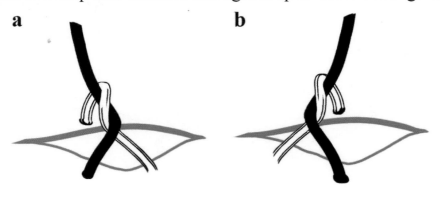

Fig. 2.21. Right and left loops (a, b)

2.5. Give the Meiss codes of the knots in Fig. 2.22, and name them.

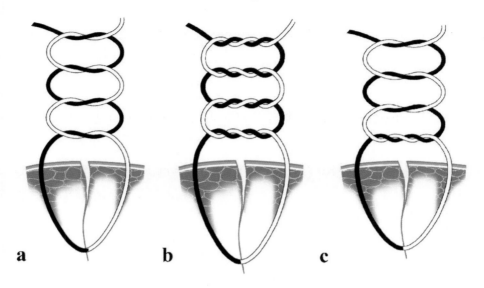

Fig. 2.22. Three different knots (a–c)

2.6. Say which loop (left or right) will be made if the end of the thread is held with the left hand? Will the way of holding the threads or of making the loop influence the direction of the loop?

2.7. Why is hand movement in making knots like the operation of a two–cylinder engine? Which of a and b in Fig. 2.23 shows the direction of hand movement in making a left loop, and which shows the direction for a right loop?

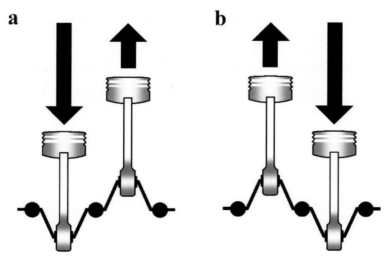

Fig. 2.23. Hand movements in loop formation (a, b)

2.8. What are the positions of the right and left hand in Fig. 2.24 – supination or pronation?

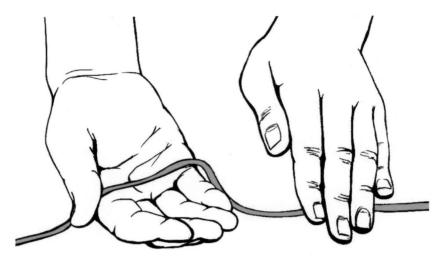

Fig. 2.24. Hands in supination and pronation

TOPIC 3.

FRONT AND REAR TECHNIQUES OF LOOP FORMATION

Techniques of loop formation

There are many ways of making loops, and various modifications of these ways. We have selected four techniques for description:

➢ **front and lower mirror** techniques, for **the end of the thread** (leading hand holds the end of the thread);

➢ **rear and lower**, for **the start of the thread** (leading hand holds the start of the thread).

Every surgeon should be proficient in the front and rear techniques of loop formation, because they can be used in any standard situation, they complement each other, and they allow the threads to be kept taut while making a second loop. However, it is worth learning several techniques, so that the student can choose which of them are most useful and then go on to master new techniques.

It is important to note that all of the explanations, which follow, are for the right hand, but by replacing every occurrence of "right" by "left", you can obtain a description for the left hand.

Steps in loop formation

Loop formation can be reduced to three steps:

- grasping and holding the threads;
- making the crossover of the threads and making the loop (the key step);
- tightening the loop.

Always make sure you carry out all steps, paying particular attention to correct grip of the threads before making each loop.

Gripping and holding the threads in front and rear loop formation

The thread grips for front and rear loop formation are similar. The difference is that, in front formation, the leading hand holds the end of the thread, while in the rear technique it holds the start of the thread.

Thread grip with the right hand. The right hand uses a frontal grip with fingers 3–4–5 ("revolver" position), while fingers 1–2 unfold freely (Fig. 3.1).

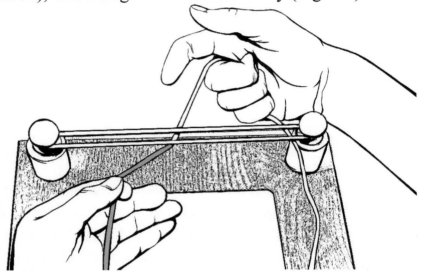

Fig. 3.1. The right hand holds the end of the thread using a frontal grip (fingers 3–4–5); the left hand holds the start of the thread with fingers 1–2.

Thread grip with the left hand. How the left hand holds the thread depends on what is most convenient in any given case, but for training purposes the student should use a grip with fingers 1–2 (Fig. 3.1) or with fingers 3–4–5 ("revolver" position).

Front technique of loop formation

There are several variants of the front technique of loop formation. Here we will explain a variant where the thread is carried by finger 1 and which is similar to the rear technique.

The front technique for the right hand, with finger 1 carrying the thread, works as follows.

Thread grip. The end of the thread is in the right hand (frontal grip with fingers 3–4–5 of the right hand), the start of the thread is in the left hand (grip with fingers 1–2).
Preparation. The right hand is pronated and the start of the thread is gripped by the distal phalange of finger 1 (Fig. 3.2).

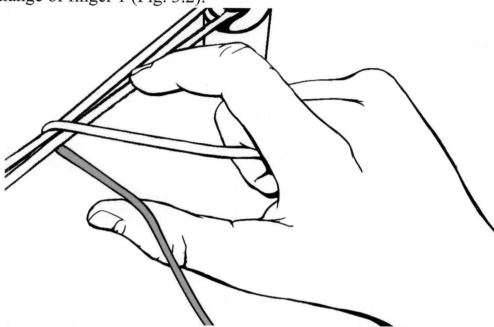

Fig. 3.2. The right hand is pronated and the start of the thread is gripped by the distal phalange of finger 1

Making the crossover. The nail of finger 1 of the right hand presses on the end of the thread (Fig. 3.3). The crossover occurs on the side of finger 1.

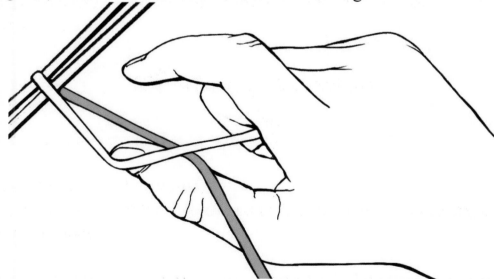

Fig. 3.3. The grip of the start of the thread is maintained, and the nail of finger 1 presses on the end of the thread. The crossover is made on the side of finger 1

Making the loop. The start of the thread is directed away from the body and laid on the end of the thread (Fig. 3.4), finger 2 of the right hand presses the start of the thread against the pad of finger 1 (Fig. 3.5). The loop is almost complete and the left hand release the start of the thread. The right hand is quickly supinated and the start of the thread is pushed into the loop (Fig. 3.6). The start of the thread is caught by the free left hand as it comes out of the loop and becomes the end of the thread (Fig. 3.7).

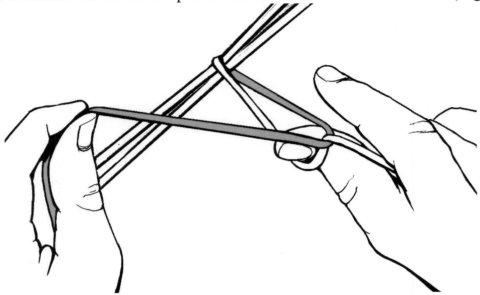

Fig. 3.4. The left hand moves the start of the thread away from the body and onto the end of the thread

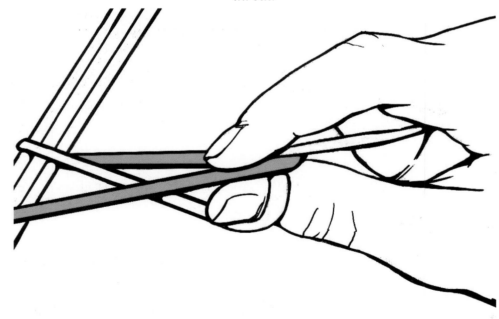

Fig. 3.5. Finger 2 of the right hand presses the start of the thread against the pad of finger 1

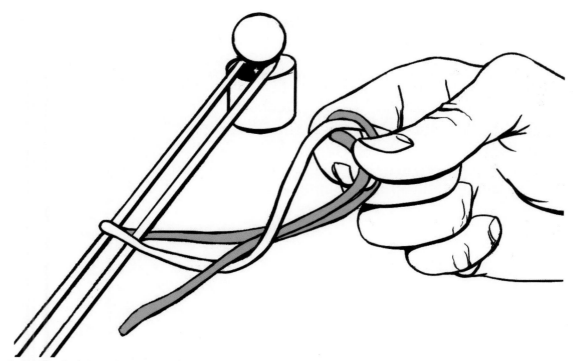

Fig. 3.6. The left hand releases the start of the thread. The right hand is supinated and the start of the thread is pushed into the loop, which has been created, by fingers 1 and 2

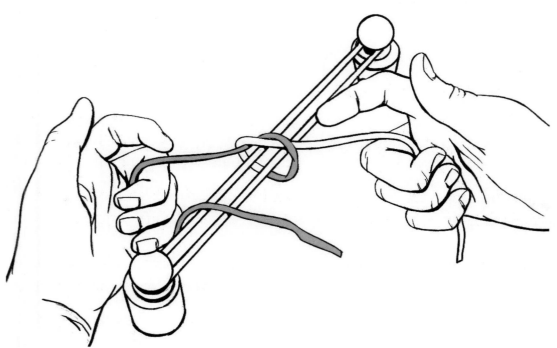

Fig. 3.7. The loop has been made. Hands and threads have changed their position

Task. Master the front technique of loop formation with the right and left hands.

Tightening of a loop

Loops must be tightened with sufficient but not excessive force.
Insufficient tightening fails to bring the tissue together, making the suture pointless. Excessive tightening constricts blood supply, which can lead to necrosis of the wound edges, and can also lead to breaking of the thread or cutting of tissue by the thread.
The best direction for tightening depends on the form of the loop and should be a natural continuation of the threads coming out of the loop (Fig. 3.8).

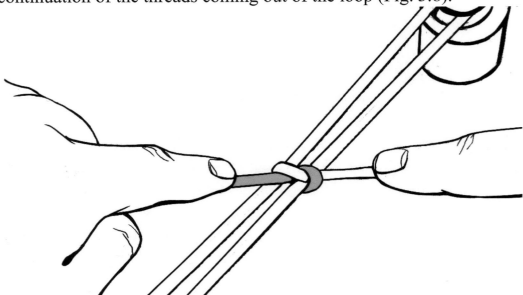

Fig. 3.8. Tightening of loops with the index finger (finger 2)

Initially loops should be tightened holding the ends of the thread with fingers 3–4–5 of the right hand and fingers 3–4–5 of the left hand and controlling tension of the threads with the index finger (finger 2). This is how it is often done in practice and transformation to other variants, when necessary, is fairly simple.
Notice particularly that tightening is carried out by the fingers and hands, and not by the whole arm. Index fingers should be placed close enough to the knot to feel the tension of the thread during tightening of the loop.
It is important not to overtighten the laces ("threads") when practicing knot formation, otherwise more time will be spent undoing knots than making them.
Task. Learn to tighten the loops with index fingers when practising the front technique of loop formation.

SELF-ASSESSMENT WHEN MAKING LOOPS

Some recommendations have already been given for self–assessment when carrying out exercises, but special remarks are in order for loops. Do not go onto the next loop–making exercise until you have achieved almost equal dexterity (smoothness, automatic movement and speed) with the right and left hands in the current exercise.

One of the main objectives of the training is to develop hand strength, so you should keep repeating earlier exercises (including match picking and exercises with the clamp).

Do not overtire your hands. It may help to practice more frequently, but reduce the duration of each practice session. Do not hurry on to the next task.

Rear technique of loop formation

The rear technique for the right hand works as follows.

Thread grip. The start of the thread is in the right hand (frontal grip with fingers 3–4–5 of the right hand), the end of the thread is in the left hand (grip with fingers 1–2).

Preparation. The right hand is pronated, finger 1 is passed under the start of the thread (Fig. 3.9) and the distal phalange touches the thread (Fig. 3.10).

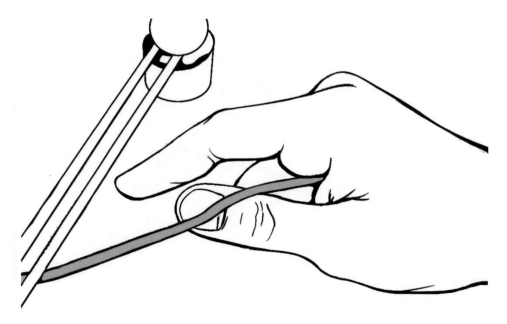

Fig. 3.9. The start of the thread is in the right hand, the right hand is pronated, and finger 1 is passed under the start of the thread

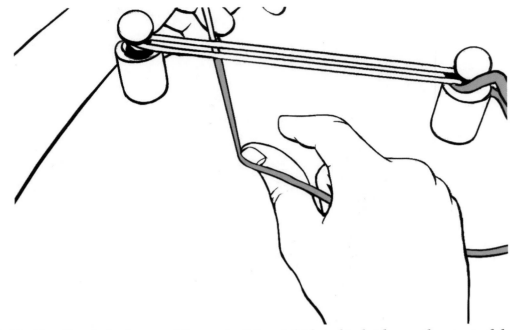

Fig. 3.10. The distal phalange of finger 1 of the right hand is laid over the start of the thread

Making the crossover. The end of the thread is laid over the start of the thread, making a crossover on the back of finger 1 of the right hand (Fig. 3.11). The pads of fingers 1 and 2 of the right hand come together (Fig. 3.12), the hand is quickly supinated, moving the front of the distal phalange of finger 2 under the crossover (Fig. 3.13).

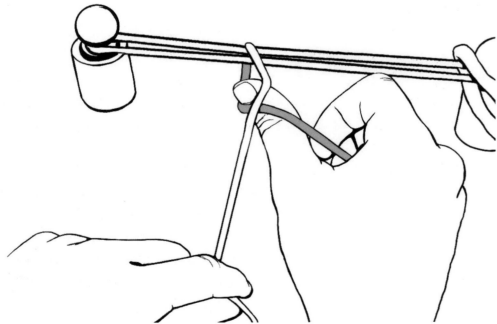

Fig. 3.11. The end of the thread is laid on the start of the thread creating the crossover on the back of finger 1 of the right hand

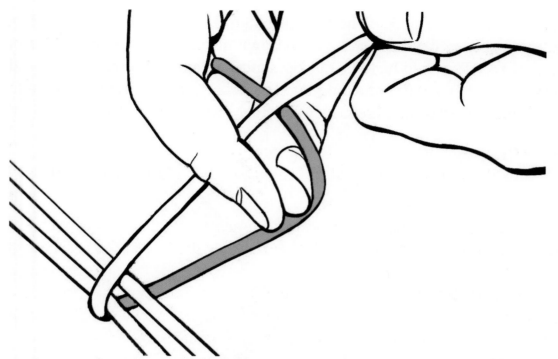

Fig. 3.12. The pads of fingers 1 and 2 of the right hand are squeezed together

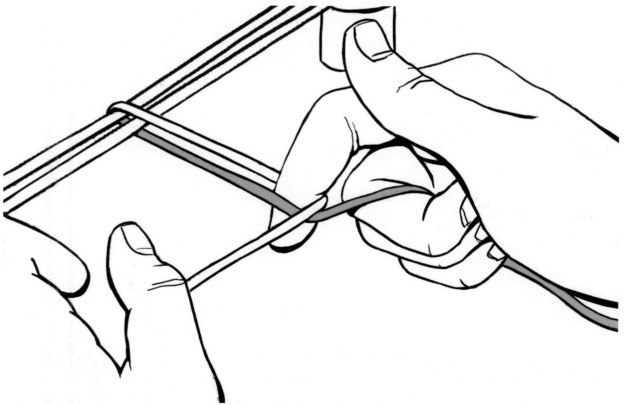

Fig. 3.13. The pad of the distal phalange of finger 2 is passed under the crossover

Making the loop. The end of the thread is laid on the pad of finger 2 (Fig. 3.14), compressed between fingers 1 and 2 of the right hand (Fig. 3.15) and pushed into the loop (Fig. 3.16). The right hand is quickly supinated and the thread is released by the left hand (Fig. 3.17). Exiting the loop, the end of the thread is caught by the left hand and becomes the start of the thread (Fig. 3.18).

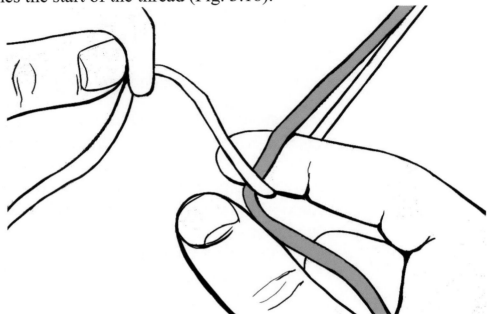

Fig. 3.14. The end of the thread on the pad of finger 2

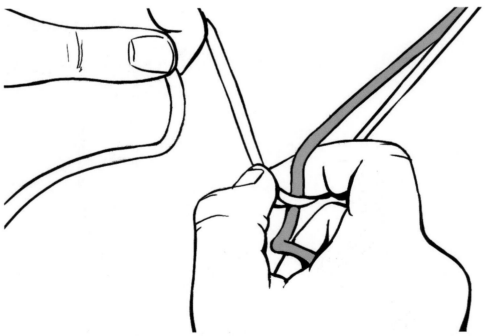

Fig. 3.15. The end of the thread is held by fingers 1 and 2 of the right hand

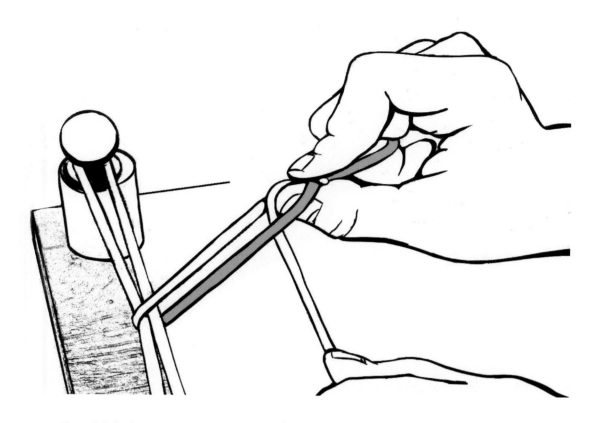

Fig. 3.16. Pronation of the hand when pushing the thread into the loop

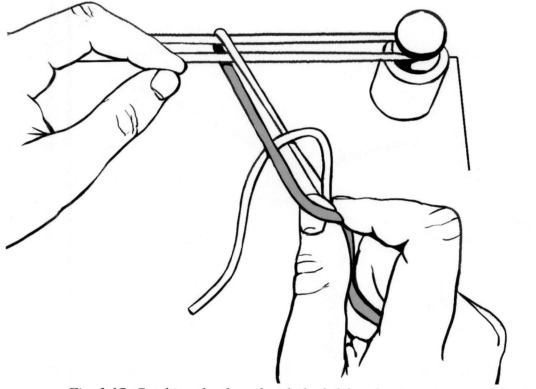

Fig. 3.17. Catching the thread with the left hand as it comes out of the loop

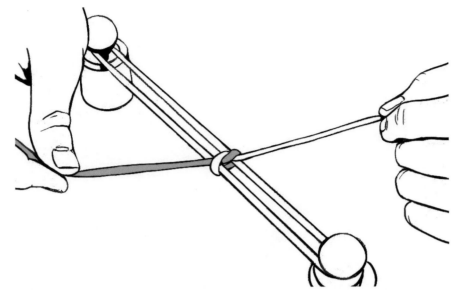

Fig. 3.18. Tightening the left loop (the end of the thread is in the right hand)

Task. Master the rear technique of loop formation with right and left hands.

Combination of front and rear techniques

In whichever hand the thread is held, if you have mastered the front and rear techniques with both hands, you can always use the front technique for the end of the thread or the rear technique for the start of the thread (Figs. 3.19, 3.20).

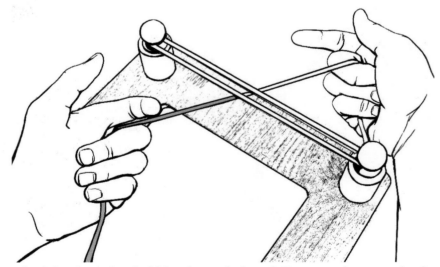

Fig. 3.19. The end of the thread is held by the right hand. You can then use the front technique for the right hand or the rear technique for the left hand. Either way, you will obtain a right loop

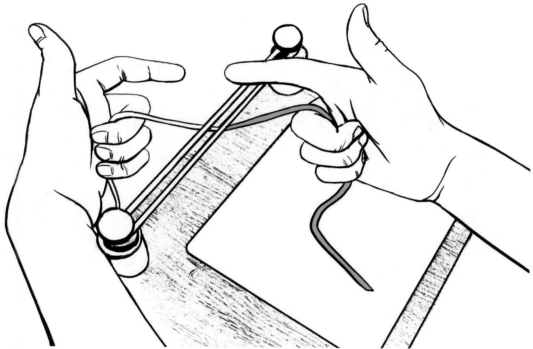

Fig. 3.20. The left hand holds the end of the thread. You can then use the front technique for the left hand or the rear technique for the right hand. Either way, you will obtain a left loop.

Once you have mastered the front and rear techniques of loop formation with the right and left hands, you can alternate right and left loops in order to make a knot correctly.

The principle of alternation between techniques in loop formation

When making a loop the threads change their status (start-end-start-end), **while remaining in the same hand, so by alternating the two techniques of loop formation** (one for the end of the thread and the other for the start), **you can make loops with the right hand alone or with the left hand alone.**

The principle of alternation is important because surgical practice mainly uses an atraumatic needle, where the thread is pressed into the eye of the needle. The needle cannot be cut off from the thread when the surgeon needs to make several knots, and that creates a risk that the surgeon will injure him/herself. Pushing the end of the thread with the needle into a loop is naturally to be avoided, since it is difficult and dangerous. Loops must therefore be made using only one end of thread (the end without the needle). This challenge can be met by alternating the loop formation techniques using

43

one hand, while always holding the other end of the thread (the end with the needle) in the other hand. In practice, this entails that the surgeon most often forms loops with the left hand.

Tasks.

1. Make loops using the right hand only, alternating the front and rear techniques.
2. Make loops using the left hand only, alternating the front and rear techniques.

TEST QUESTIONS AND TASKS

3.1. What is the name of the thread grip shown in Fig. 3.21? Is this grip used to make loops with the front or the rear technique?

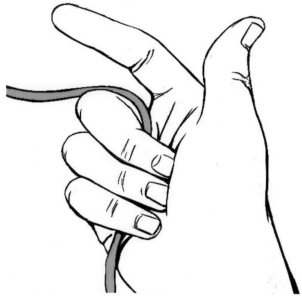

Fig. 3.21. Thread grip with the right hand

3.2. Which loop is made by which technique (front or rear) using the thread grip shown in Fig. 3.22?

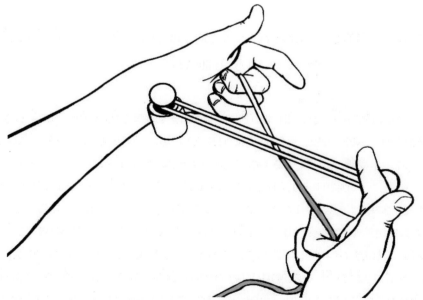

Fig. 3.22. Thread grip before loop formation on the training apparatus

3.3. Add the missing second step in loop formation:
   1) grasp and hold the threads;

2) …;
3) tighten the loops.

3.4. Identify the type of loop (simple or complex, right or left) which is being tightened in Fig. 3.23. Is the loop being tightened correctly?

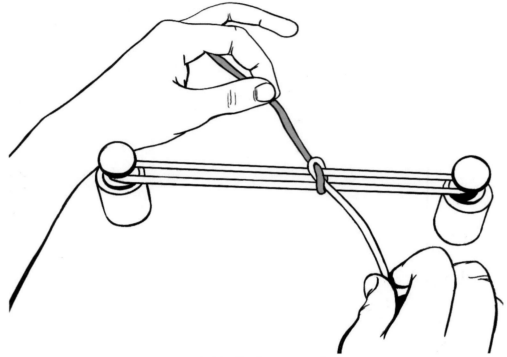

Fig. 3.23. Tightening a loop

3.5. State the principle of alternation of techniques and explain its importance.

TOPIC 4.

USE OF A CLAMP IN THE FRONT AND REAR TECHNIQUES OF LOOP FORMATION

It should be noted that one hand always dominates when forming loops, while the other only holds the thread (for example, with a frontal grip using fingers–1 and –2).

When alternating the front and rear techniques of loop formation using only the left hand, grip of the thread with the right hand can easily be replaced by a grip using a surgical clamp held by the right hand.

Therefore, when holding the thread with a clamp, you need to be able to form loops with the left hand alone.

It is important to note that you need to bring the index finger closer to the knot in order to tighten loops when using a clamp.

Advice to left-handed students: all surgical instruments are made for right-handed people, so people who are left-handed need to develop their right hand and accustom their right hand to work with surgical instruments.

Advice to right-handed students: situations where you need to make a loop with the left hand occur regularly in surgical practice and often coincide with other difficult circumstances, so it is important to develop the left hand.

Front and rear techniques of loop formation with the left hand using a surgical clamp

The sequence of movements for the front and rear techniques of loop formation using the left hand are almost identical, with and without a surgical clamp.

Recommendations. If difficulties arise when making loops by the front or rear technique using the left hand, try the same technique using the right hand. If difficulties arise when making loops by the front or rear technique using a clamp in the right hand, try the same technique using the left hand, but without a clamp.

Notice that the thread grips for loop formation using the front and rear techniques with the left hand and surgical clamp are similar.

The thread is held in a frontal grip by fingers 3–4–5 of the left hand, fingers 1–2 are unfolded and loose ("revolver" position).

It will be found most convenient to hold the clamp with fingers 1–3 of the right hand.

Front technique for the left hand using a clamp

The front technique for the left hand using a clamp works as follows.

Thread grip. The end of the thread is in the left hand (frontal grip with fingers 3–4–5); the start of the thread is held by the clamp in the right hand.

Preparation. The left hand is pronated, the start of the thread is gripped by the distal phalange of finger 1 (Fig. 4.1).

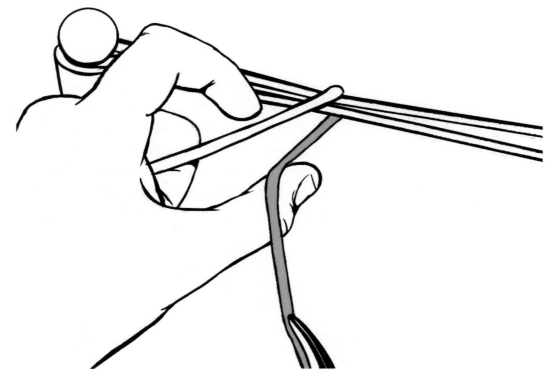

Fig. 4.1. The left hand is pronated; finger 1 grips the start of the thread with the distal phalange

Making the crossover. The nail of finger 1 is laid onto the end of the thread (Fig. 4.2). The crossover is made on the side of finger 1 of the left hand.

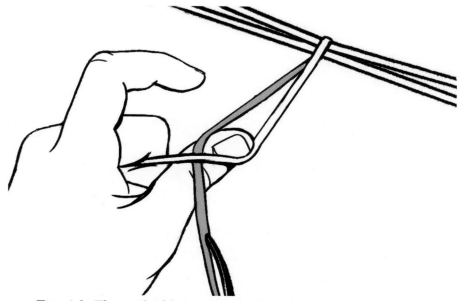

Fig. 4.2. The nail of finger 1 is laid onto the end of the thread

Making the loop. The start of the thread is directed away from the body and laid onto the end of the thread (Fig. 4.3); finger 2 of the left hand presses the start of the thread onto the pad of finger 1 (Fig. 4.4). The loop is nearly made and the clamp releases the start of the thread. The left hand is rapidly supinated and the start of the thread is pushed into the loop (Fig. 4.5). Coming out of the loop, the start of the thread is gripped by the clamp and tightened by the loop. The thread in in the left hand now becomes the start of the thread, and the rear technique using the left hand can be initiated.

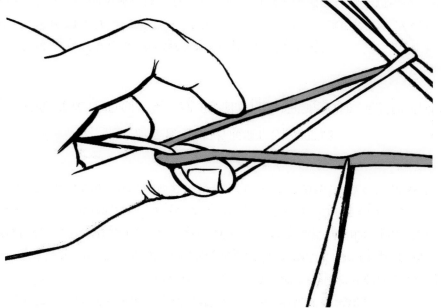

Fig. 4.3. The start of the thread is directed away from the body and laid onto the end of the thread

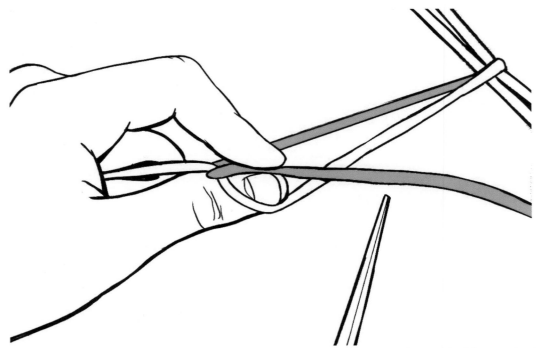

Fig. 4.4. Finger 2 of the left hand presses the start of the thread onto the pad of finger 1, the clamp is released and the start of the thread is pushed into the loop

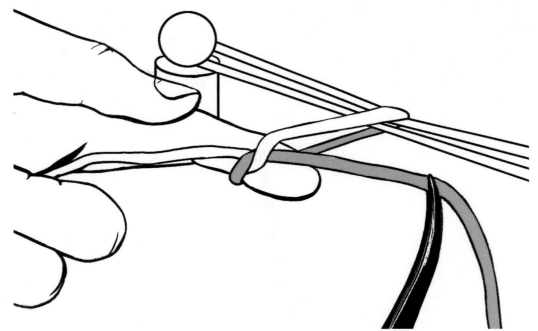

Fig. 4.5. The loop has been made. The clamp again grips the start of the thread, which becomes the end of the thread

Task. Master the front technique of loop formation with the left hand using a clamp in the right hand.

Rear technique for the left hand using a clamp

The rear technique for the left hand using a clamp works as follows.

Thread grip. The start of the thread is in the left hand (frontal grip with fingers 3–4–5), the end of the thread is held by the clamp in the right hand.

Preparation. The left hand is pronated; the distal phalange of finger 1 of the left hand is laid onto the start of the thread (Fig. 4.6).

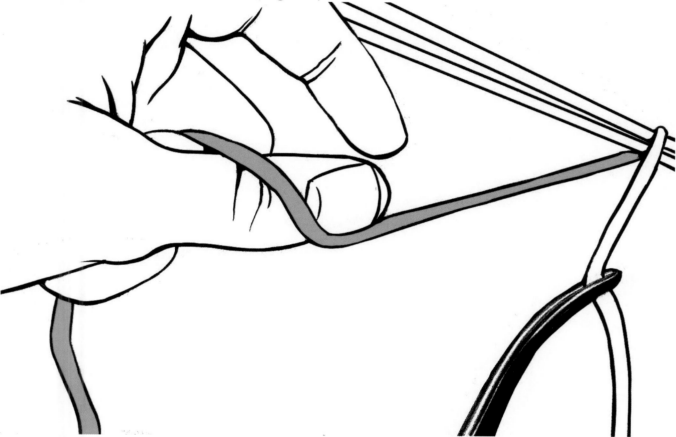

Fig. 4.6. The start of the thread is in the left hand, the left hand is pronated, the distal phalange of finger 1 of the left hand is laid onto the start of the thread.

Making the crossover. The end of the thread is laid onto the start of the thread, making the crossover on the back of finger 1 of the left hand (Fig. 4.7). Fingers 1–2 of the left hand are folded and the hand is rapidly supinated, moving the front of the distal phalange of finger 2 under the crossover (Fig. 4.8).

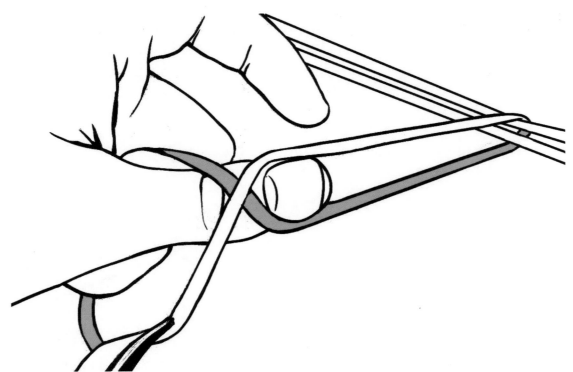

Fig. 4.7. The end of the thread is laid onto the start, making the crossover on the back of finger 1 of the left hand

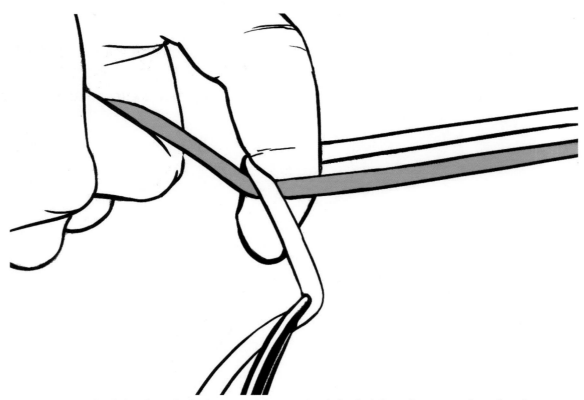

Fig. 4.8. The pad of the distal phalange of finger 2 of the left hand is moved under the crossover

Making the loop. The end of the thread is laid onto the pad of finger 2 (Fig. 4.8), fingers 1–2 of the left hand grasp the thread (Fig. 4.9) and push it into the loop, the left hand is rapidly pronated and the clamp releases the thread. Coming out of the loop, the end of the thread is grasped by the clamp and becomes start of the thread (Fig. 4.10).

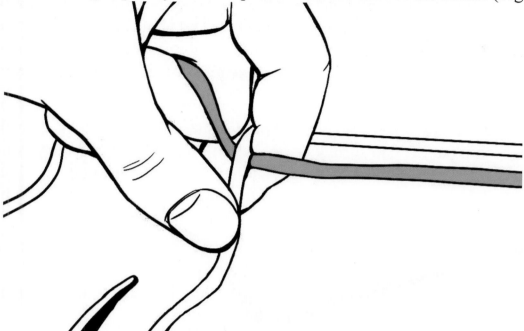

Fig. 4.9. Fingers 1–2 of the left hand grip the end of the thread

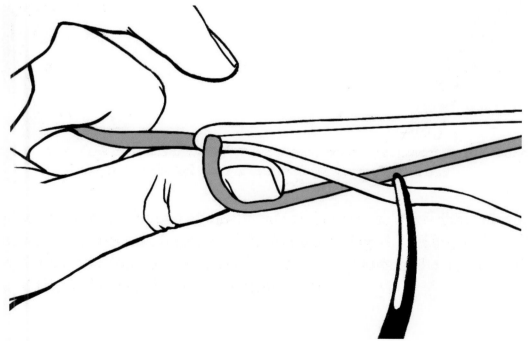

Fig. 4.10. After passing through the loop, the thread is again grasped by the clamp

Tasks. 1. Master the rear technique of loop formation with the left hand using a surgical clamp in the right hand.

2. Make loops with the left hand, alternating the front and rear techniques and holding the thread with the right hand using a clamp. This skill is very important in the operating theatre and should be practised until it becomes second nature.

Summary

Knots consist of loops, which can be right or left, simple or complex. It is sufficient to know one technique of loop formation in order to make knots correctly, since each technique enables formation of both right and left loops. If the end of the thread is in the right hand, a right loop will be made. If the end of the thread is in the left hand, a left loop will be made. Right and left loops always alternate $(+ - + -)$.

When loops are being made correctly, the motion of the hands resembles the work of a two–cylinder engine. The same thread is alternately the start and the end of the thread, but is held all the time in the same hand. The thread is not passed from hand to hand, but remains all the time in the hand, which initially grasped it.

One hand leads the formation of loops. In the front technique, it is the hand that holds the end of the thread, and in the rear technique, it is the hand that holds the start of the thread.

Remember to make sure that the training apparatus is positioned in a way that makes it easy to carry out the exercises.

Loops are tightened following the natural direction of the thread. Loops must not be tightened with twisting of the thread (Fig. 4.11).

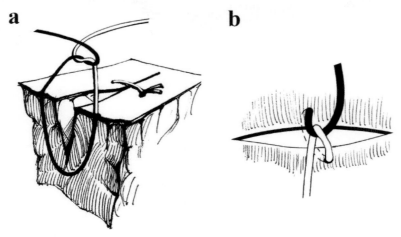

Fig. 4.11. Loop formation with twisting of the threads (a, b)

TEST QUESTIONS AND TASKS

4.1. Compare loop formation with and without a clamp, using the front and rear techniques. Describe the benefits of using a clamp. Which way of making a loop is the quickest?

4.2. How does the use of a clamp save thread when making knots (Fig. 4.12)?

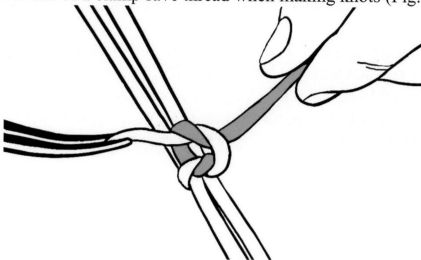

Fig. 4.12. Use of a clamp to make a square knot

4.3. Describe the specific features of loop tightening using a clamp (Fig. 4.13).

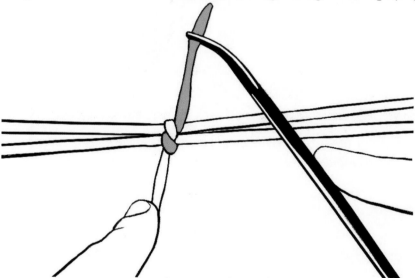

Fig. 4.13. Tightening a loop using a clamp

TOPIC 5.

MAKING A COMPLEX LOOP BY THE FRONT AND REAR TECHNIQUES

Second loop

It is important to tension the threads in the second loop correctly in order to preserve the first loop (Fig. 5.1). The second loop is important because, in combination with the first loop, it forms the knot.

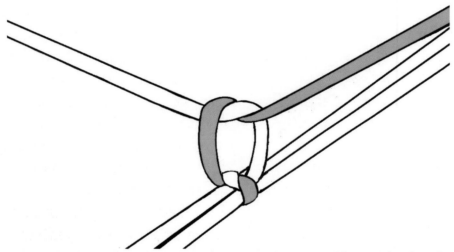

Fig. 5.1. Tensioning of the threads when tightening the second loop. The first loop has been tightened (the tubes of the training apparatus meet)

When a knot is being made, tissues are pulled tight, and tension must be applied to both threads and tissues. When adequate tension has been obtained, both front and rear techniques are perfectly suitable for making the second loop, since they allow the thread to be kept under tension from tightening of the first loop until tightening of the second, preventing the first loop from coming undone during this time.

A complex loop may be appropriate if the tissues exert much resistance when they are being brought together by a suture, since a complex loop makes the knot stronger. The complex loop is part of the structure of the academic and surgeon's knots.

Front technique of complex loop formation

The making of complex loops using the front and rear techniques is a two–step technique. All the initial stages of complex loop formation by the front and rear techniques are identical to the making of simple loops by the two techniques. The differences occur only in the last stage.

The first four steps are identical to the front technique of loop formation:

- **Thread grip.**
- **Preparation.**
- **Making the crossover**.

Making the loop. Grasp the start of the thread with the free left hand as it comes out of the loop, but do not tighten the thread (Fig. 5.2).

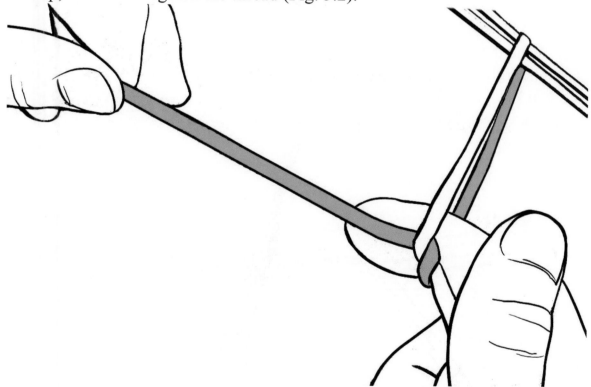

Fig. 5.2. A simple right loop has been made but not tightened

Making the complex loop. The operation essentially repeats the making of the first loop in step 4 above. Finger 1 of the right hand returns to where it was before the making of the first loop (Fig. 5.3).

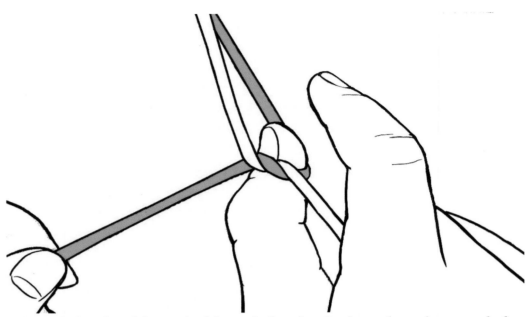

Fig. 5.3. The right hand and finger 1 of the right hand go back to where they were before the first loop was made

The start of the thread is again laid against the pad of finger 1 and gripped by finger 2 (Fig. 5.4), the right hand is rapidly supinated and the start of the thread is again pushed into the loop (Fig. 5.5). The start of the thread becomes the end of the thread. A right–double complex loop is made (+2) (Fig. 5.6).

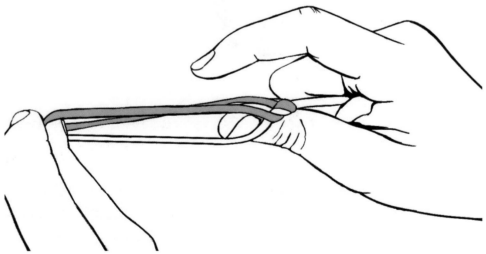

Fig. 5.4. The start of the thread is again laid onto the pad of finger 1 and gripped by finger 2

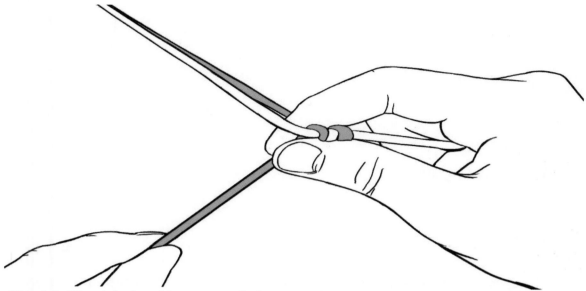

Fig. 5.5. The right hand is supinated, the start of the thread is pushed into the loop again

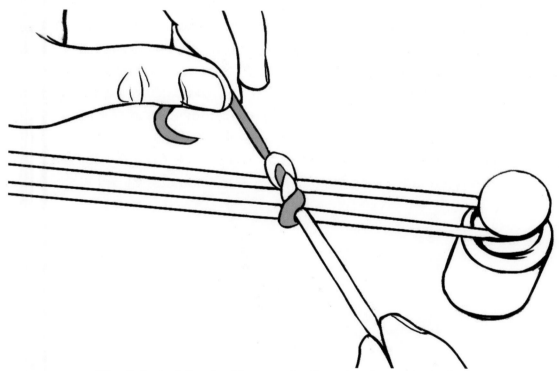

Fig. 5.6. A right–double complex loop has been made (+2)

Task. Make a complex loop, +2 and –2, using the front technique.

Rear technique of complex loop formation

The first four steps are identical to the rear technique of loop formation:

- **Thread grip.**
- **Preparation.**
- **Making the crossover.**

Making the loop. Grasp the end of the thread with the free left hand as it comes out of the loop, but do not tighten the loop.

Making the complex loop. The operation simply repeats the previous stage (making the loop). Finger 2 of the right hand returns to where it was before the formation of the first loop (Fig. 5.7), the end of the thread is again laid onto the pad of finger 2 (Fig. 5.8) and held by fingers 1–2 (Fig. 5.9), the right hand is quickly pronated and the thread is pushed into the loop (Fig. 5.10). The left–double complex loop (–2) is then complete.

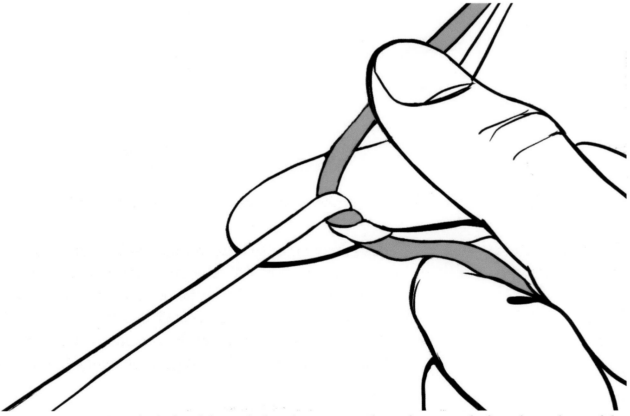

Fig. 5.7. Finger 2 and whole of the right hand return to where they were before the making of the first loop

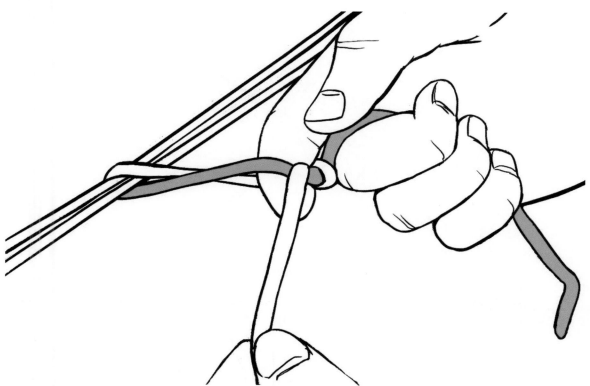

Fig. 5.8. The end of the thread is again laid onto the pad of finger 2

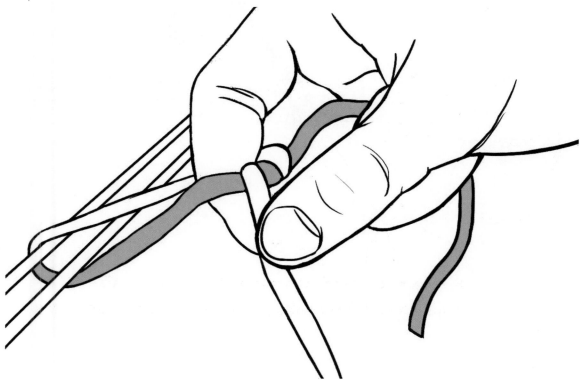

Fig. 5.9. The end of the thread is held between fingers 1–2

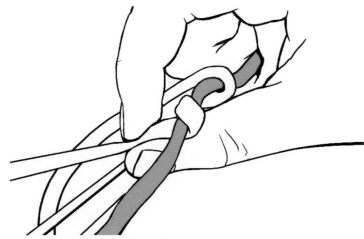

Fig. 5.10. The end of the thread is pushed through the loop, the left–double complex loop (–2) is complete

Task. Make complex loop +2 and –2 using the rear technique.

TEST QUESTIONS AND TASKS

5.1. What is the importance of the second loop in a knot?

5.2. What prevents the first loop coming undone before the second loop has been tightened and the knot has been made (Fig. 5.11)?

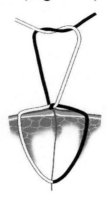

Fig. 5.11. Tightening of the second loop

5.3. Which knot has a structure with one complex loop? Which knot (square, surgeon's or academic) consists only of complex loops?

5.4. Practise the front and rear techniques of loop formation using a clamp. Hold the thread with the clamp in the right hand. Is there much difference between making simple and complex loops using a clamp?

TOPIC 6.

LOWER AND LOWER MIRROR TECHNIQUES OF LOOP FORMATION

The lower mirror technique is designed for the end of the thread (the leading hand is the hand that holds the end of the thread), **while the lower technique is for the start of the thread** (the leading hand is the hand that holds the start of the thread).
Practise each stage of loop formation:

- **Gripping and holding the threads.**
- **Making the crossover and the loop.**
- **Tightening the loop.**

Make sure that you are holding the threads correctly before making each loop. All of the explanations, which are given, are for the right hand.

Lower mirror technique

The lower mirror technique of loop formation works as follows.
Thread grip. The right hand grasps the end of the thread between the pads of fingers 1–3 (Fig. 6.1). The start of the thread is held between the pads of fingers 1–2 of the left hand.

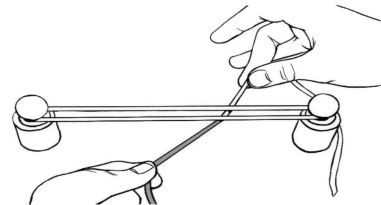

Fig. 6.1. The end of the thread is held by fingers 1–3 of the right hand

Preparation. The right hand is supinated, finger 2 is passed under the end of the thread, and the thread is laid onto the finger near first interphalangeal joint (Fig. 6.2). The start of the thread is brought to the same place from beneath.

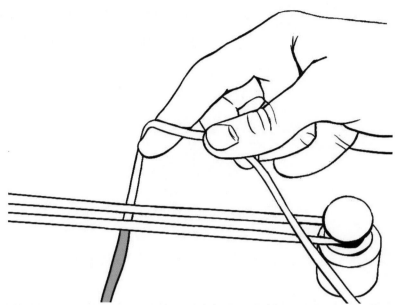

Fig. 6.2. Supination of the right hand and positioning of finger 2 under the end of the thread

Making the crossover. The start of the thread is directed away from the body and laid over the end of the thread, making the crossover on the side of finger 2 of the right hand (Fig. 6.3).

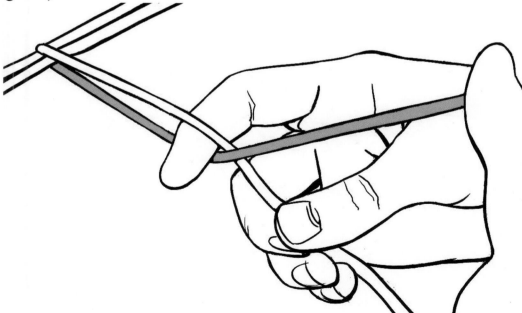

Fig. 6.3. Crossover of the threads on the side of finger 2 of the right hand

Making the loop. Finger 2 of the right hand is bent around the start of the thread. The nail of finger 2 catches the end of the thread (Fig. 6.4). Finger 2 unbends, pulling the thread into the loop (Fig. 6.5). At the same time fingers 1–3 of the right hand relax and the end of the thread is gripped by the sides of fingers 2–3 (Fig. 6.6). Coming out of the loop, the end of the thread becomes the start of the thread.

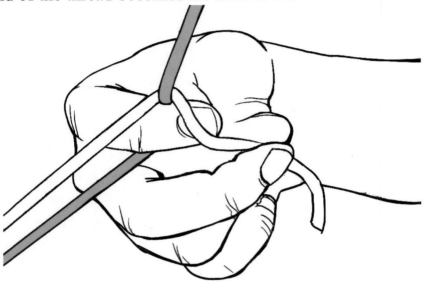

Fig. 6.4. Finger 2 of the right hand is bent around the start of the thread. The nail of finger 2 catches the end of the thread

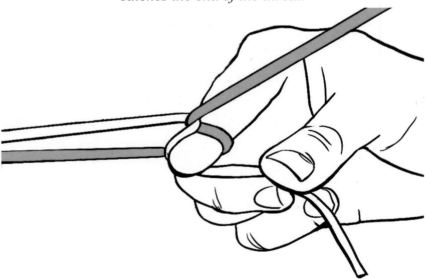

Fig. 6.5. Finger 2 of the right hand is unbent, pulling the end of the thread into the loop, and the end of the thread is gripped by the sides of fingers 2–3

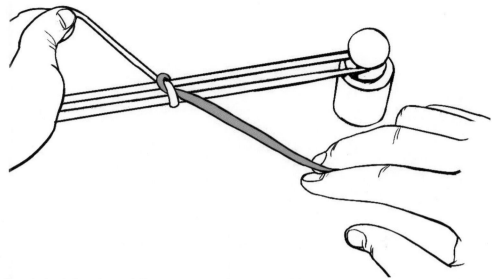

Fig. 6.6. The end of the thread becomes the start of the thread. It remains in the right hand and is held between the sides of fingers 2–3. A right loop is made

Task. Practise loop formation using the lower mirror technique with the right and left hands.

Lower technique

The lower technique of loop formation works as follows.
Thread grip. The start of the thread is in the right hand. The two hands grip the threads in the same way, compressing them between the pads of the distal phalanges of fingers 1–2 (Fig. 6.7).

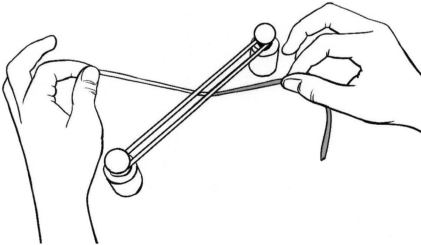

Fig. 6.7. The start and end of the thread is held by fingers 1–2

Preparation. Fingers 3–4–5 of the right hand are pressed together, the hand is rapidly supinated, finger 5 is laid onto the start of the thread (Fig. 6.8).

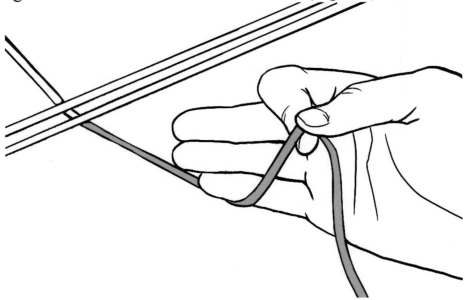

Fig. 6.8. The right hand is supinated, fingers 3–4–5 are pressed together, finger 5 is laid on the start of the thread.

Making the crossover. The end of the thread is brought down, touching finger 3 of the right hand, and laid onto the start of the thread, making the crossover in the air adjacent to finger 4 of the right hand (Fig. 6.9).

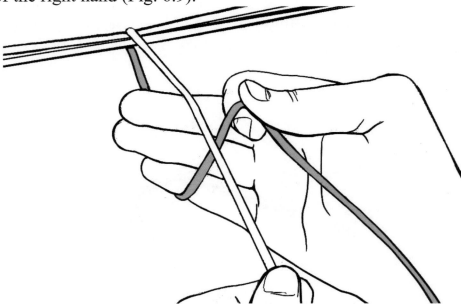

Fig. 6.9. The end of the thread touches finger 3 and makes the crossover in the air adjacent to finger 4 of the right hand

Making the loop. Finger 3 of the right hand bends and catches the end of the thread, and the fingernail passes under the start of the thread (Fig. 6.10). Finger 3 unbends, catches the start of the thread with the nail, and the start of the thread is gripped between the sides of fingers 3–4 (Fig. 6.11). At the same time, fingers 1–2 of the right hand unbend and release the thread. The start of the thread is pulled into the loop and becomes the end of the thread (Fig. 6.12).

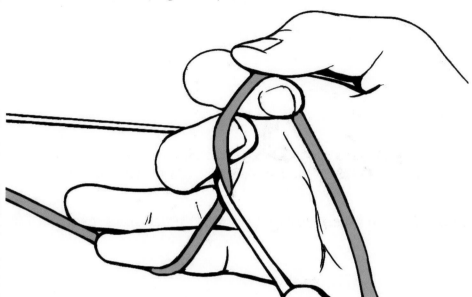

Fig. 6.10. Finger 3 of the right hand is bent and the fingernail is passed under the start of the thread

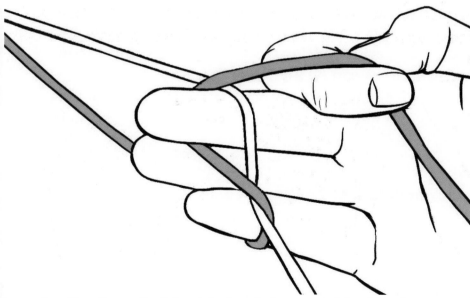

Fig. 6.11. After unbending finger 3 of the right hand, the start of the thread is gripped by the sides of fingers 3–4 of the right hand

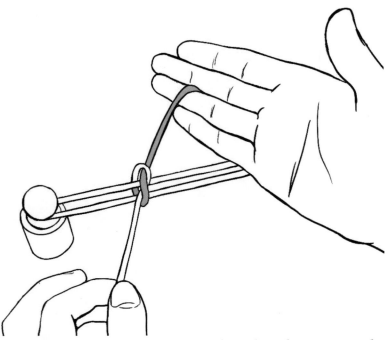

Fig. 6.12. The start of the thread has become the end of the thread, and remains in the right hand. It is still gripped between the sides of fingers 3–4. A left loop has been made.

Task. Practise making loops using the lower technique with the right and left hands.

Alternation of loop formation techniques

The front and lower mirror techniques of loop formation are meant for the end of the thread, while the rear and lower techniques are meant for the start of the thread, so the techniques can be alternated.

The role of the hands alternates when making loops – each hand takes turns holding the start and end of the thread. Therefore, it is possible to tie knots, using one of the following approaches:

- **using one technique, but alternating the hands;**
- **using one hand, but alternating the techniques:**
  - ✓ front – rear,
  - ✓ front – lower,
  - ✓ lower mirror – rear,
  - ✓ lower mirror – lower.

Tasks. 1. Make loops using the right hand only, alternating the front, rear, lower mirror and lower techniques. 2. Make loops using only the left hand, alternating the front, rear, lower mirror and lower techniques.

It is important to keep repeating earlier exercises. Some exercises can take a month of training before they become automatic, and they can easily be forgotten thereafter unless they are practiced.

The single-step technique of complex loop formation

The originality of this technique is that both hands play an equal part, so that a complex loop is obtained "in one movement". We describe it here for the sake of comparison with the two–step techniques described above. Before starting, the student should again practise making right and left loops with the lower mirror technique.

Thread grip. The end of the thread is in the right hand. The two ends of the thread are gripped in the same way – between the pads of fingers 1–3 of the two hands (Fig. 6.13).

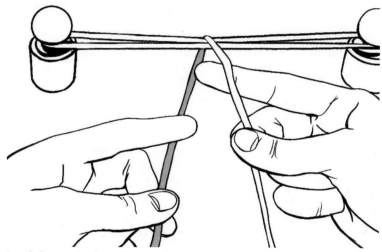

Fig. 6.13. Finger 2 of the right hand is under the end of the thread. Finger 2 of the left hand is above the start of the thread

Preparation. Finger 2 of the right hand is under the end of the thread, finger 2 of the left hand is above the start of the thread (Fig. 6.13).

Making the crossover. The start of the thread is caught from above by bending of finger 2 of the right hand, and the end of the thread is caught from below by bending of finger 2 of the left hand. The crossover of the threads then hangs in the air between the hands (Fig. 6.14).

71

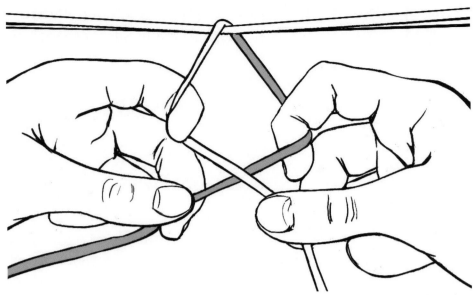

Fig. 6.14. The start of the thread is caught by bending of finger 2 of the right hand, and the end of the thread is caught by bending of finger 2 of the left hand. The crossover hangs in the air

Making the complex loop. The distal phalange of finger 2 of the right hand pulls up the end of the thread and drives it into the loop, and the distal phalange of finger 2 of the left hand does the same with the start of the thread (Fig. 6.15). The threads are pulled into the loop by finger 2 of each hand and grasped by the sides of fingers 2–3 (Fig. 6.16).

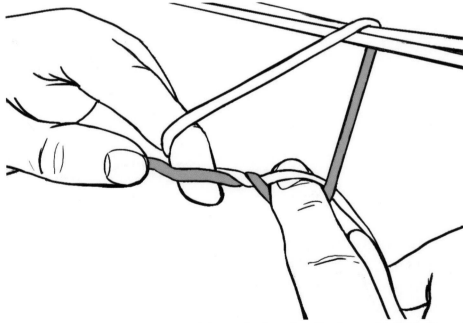

Fig. 6.15. The distal phalange of finger 2 of the right hand pulls the end of the thread into the loop, while the distal phalange of finger 2 of the left hand does the same for the start of the thread

72

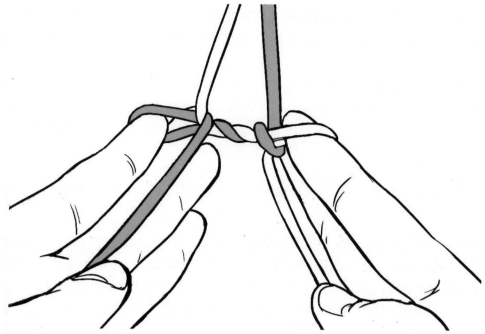

Fig. 6.16. Transition to grip of the threads by the sides of fingers 2–3 when pulling the threads into the loop

This advanced technique is worth learning because it helps to develop coordination between the two hands, but it is hardly ever used in practice because of temporary loss of control over tension of the threads and the difficulty of the technique when wearing gloves.

Task. Make a complex loop (+2 and –2) using the technique described above.

TEST QUESTIONS AND TASKS

6.1. Which loop–making techniques would be possible in Fig. 6.17.

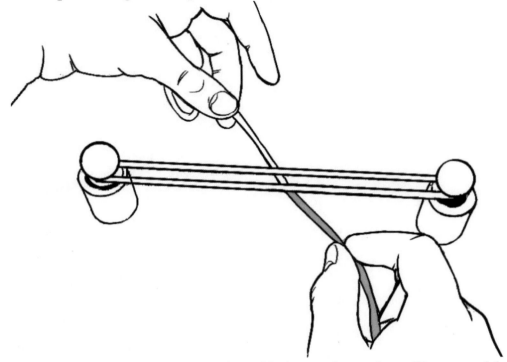

Fig. 6.17. Grip of the start and end of the thread before making a loop. The start of the thread is in the right hand, held by fingers 1–2, the end of the thread is in the left hand, held by fingers 1–3

6.2. Explain the choice of loop–making techniques, using Table 6.1.

	Left Hand	Right Hand
End of the thread	**Front or lower mirror technique**	
Start of the thread	**Rear or lower technique**	

Table 6.1. Choice of loop–making techniques

6.3. Hold one end of the thread using a clamp in the right hand, as shown in Fig. 6.18. Is it or is it not possible from this position to make a square knot using only the left hand by a combination of the lower and lower mirror techniques?

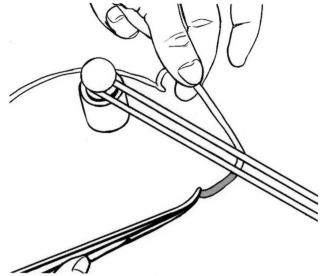

Fig. 6.18. The end of the thread is in the left hand; a clamp in the right hand holds the start of the thread

6.4. Compare your muscle sensations when you hold the threads under tension in order to make the second loop by the techniques described above (lower, lower mirror, front and rear). Are all of the techniques equally good at maintaining tension of the threads over the first loop when making the second loop?

6.5. Repeat the two–step formation of complex loops using the front and rear techniques. What basic differences are there between the two techniques? Put on medical gloves (make sure they are a good fit) and compare the techniques again.

TOPIC 7.

LOOP CREATION BY THE WIND-AROUND METHOD

The wind-around method using a surgical clamp

We will focus on how to make loops and knots by the wind-around method with a clamp and with the right hand, since in most cases the clamp is held in the right hand. **A right loop is made as follows.**

Thread grip. The left hand holds the start of the thread with a pressure grip between Fingers 1–2. The end of the thread is free (Fig. 7.1).

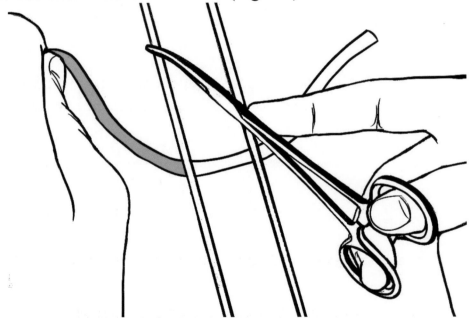

Fig. 7.1. The start of the thread is in the left hand, the clamp is between the start and end of the thread

Preparation. Be sure to position the clamp between start and end of the thread (see Fig. 7.1).

Making the loop. Put the start of the thread on the clamp. Wind the start of the thread around the clamp once (Fig. 7.2). Catch the end of the thread with the clamp (Fig. 7.3.)

and pull it towards you with the clamp. It then becomes the start of the thread and a right loop has been made (Fig. 7.4).

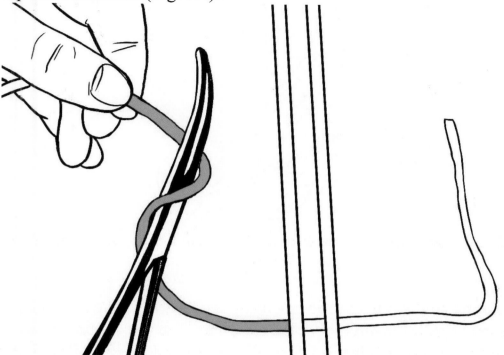

Fig. 7.2. The start of the thread wound once around the clamp

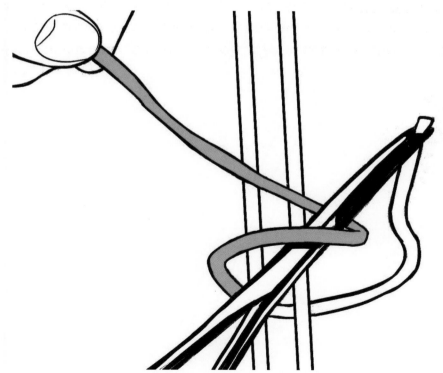

Fig. 7.3. The end of the thread caught by the clamp

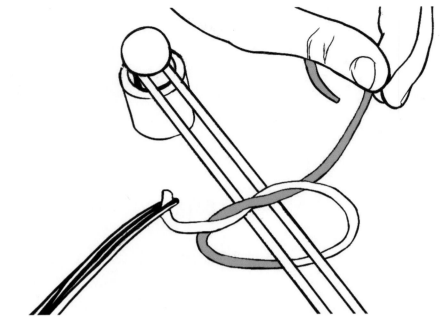

Fig. 7.4. A right loop has been made. The end of the thread becomes the start

A left loop is made as follows.
Thread grip. The start of the thread is released from the clamp, the left hand continues to hold the end of the thread (Fig. 7.5).

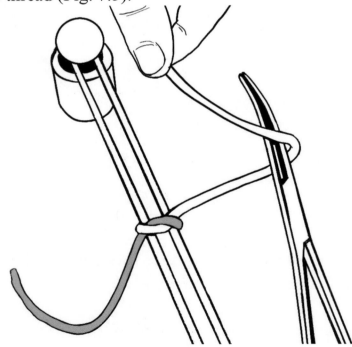

Fig. 7.5. The clamp is between the start and end of the thread. The end of the thread is brought over the clamp

Preparation. The clamp is between the start and end of the thread (see Fig. 7.5). **Making the loop**. The end of the thread is brought over the clamp (see Fig. 7.5) and wound once around the clamp (Fig. 7.6). The start of the thread is caught by the clamp (Fig. 7.7), pulled away from you and becomes the end of the thread. A left loop has been made (Fig. 7.8).

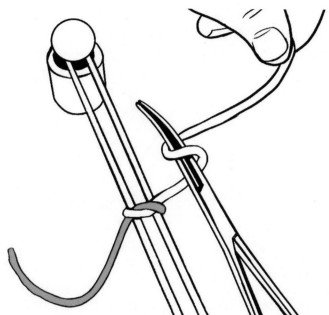

Fig. 7.6. The end of the thread wound around the clamp

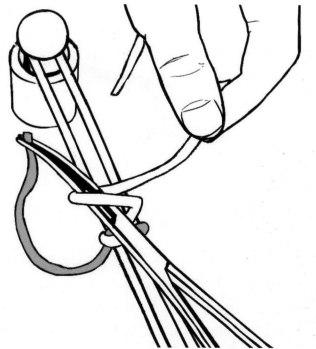

Fig. 7.7. The start of the thread caught by the clamp

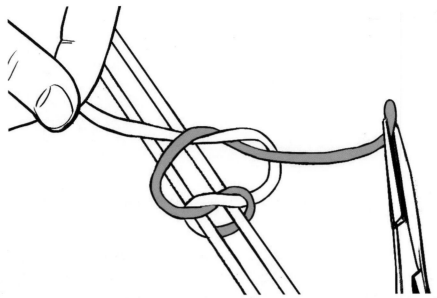

Fig. 7.8. The thread is pulled into the loop by the clamp. A left loop has been made

It is important to note that loops made using the wind-around method follow the same rules as loops made by other methods. The rule that the hand holding the end of the thread determines whether the loop is left or right also applies, but here it can be rephrased: if the clamp catches the end of the thread, a right loop is made; if the clamp catches the start of the thread, a left loop is made.

Task. Make right and left loops using the wind-around method with a surgical clamp.

Making complex loops with a surgical clamp by the wind–around method

The only difference between a single and a double wind-around loop is that, in the latter, the thread is wound around the clamp twice instead of once.

A double right loop is made as follows.

Thread grip. The end of the thread is free, the start of the thread is held by the left hand (most conveniently, by fingers 1–2).

Preparation. The clamp is between the start and end of the thread, the start of the thread is laid over the clamp.

Making the loop. The start of the thread is wound around the clamp twice (Fig. 7.9). The clamp catches the end of the thread, pulls it towards you, and the end becomes the start. The double right loop is tightened (Fig. 7.10).

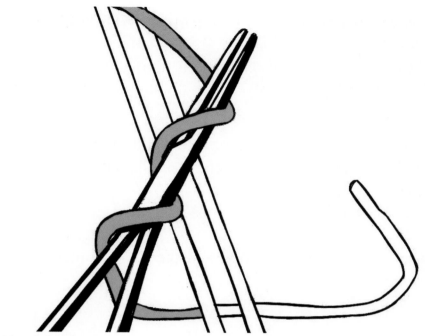

Fig. 7.9. The start of the thread is wound around the clamp twice

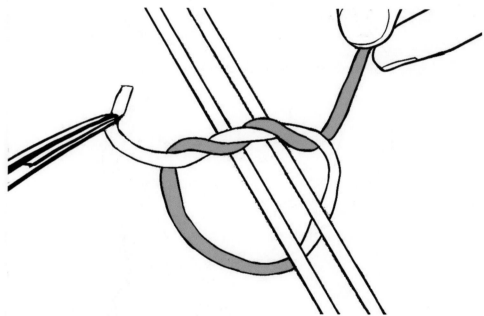

Fig. 7.10. The thread is pulled into the loop by the clamp. The double right loop is tightened

Task. Make right and left double loops by the wind-around method with a surgical clamp.

Use of two clamps to make loops with a short thread

Two clamps can be used to make loops with a short thread as follows.

Preparation. Use a 10-15 cm section of the lace and two surgical clamps (held by fingers 1–3).

Thread grip. The end of the thread is free. The right-hand clamp grips the tip of the start of the thread (the thread is effectively "lengthened" by this attachment of the clamp) (Fig. 7.11).

Preparation. The left-hand clamp is positioned between the start and end of the thread (see Fig. 7.11).

Making the loop. Both clamps are used and the loop is made by the wind-around method (Fig. 7.11 and 7.12).

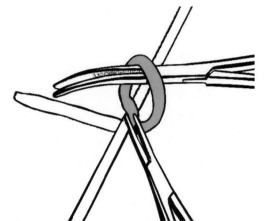

Fig. 7.11. The start of the thread is wound once around the clamp

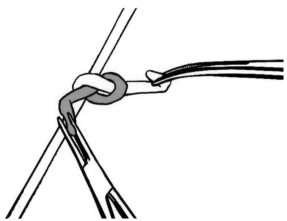

Fig. 7.12. The right loop is tightened

Task. Make right and left loops with short threads by the wind-around method using two surgical clamps.

TEST QUESTIONS AND TASKS

7.1. State the rules for making loops by the wind-around method with a clamp.

7.2. In Fig. 7.13 something has gone wrong in the making of a wind-around loop. What is it?

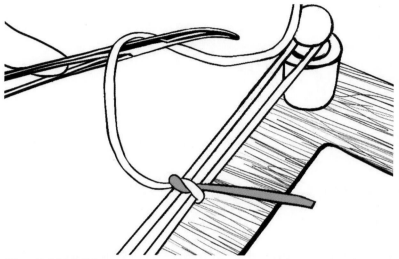

Fig. 7.13. Making a second loop by the wind-around method

7.3. Repeat the front and rear methods of loop making with a clamp in the right hand. Take a 10-15 cm lace. Practise making loops with a short thread by the front and rear methods using two clamps. Use Figs. 7.14, 7.15 and 7.16 for visual guidance. Note how the left-hand clamp serves to "lengthen" the thread. Judge whether or not this method suits you.

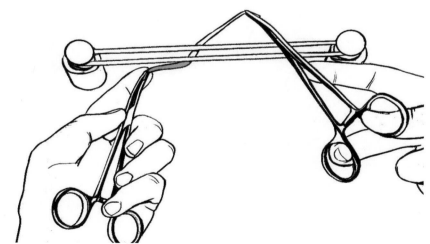

Fig. 7.14. A short thread is "lengthened" by the left-hand clamp

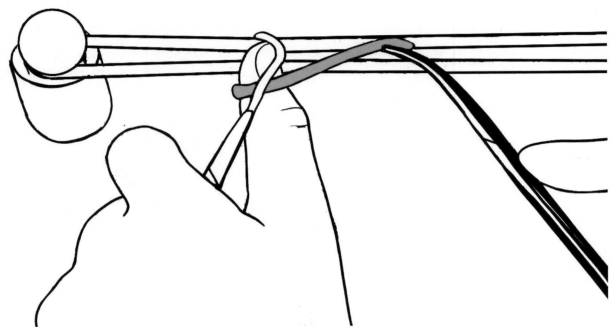

Fig. 7.15. Thread crossover when making a loop by the front method using two clamps on a short thread

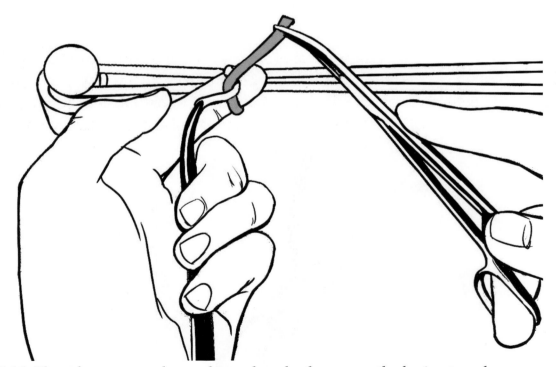

Fig. 7.16. Thread crossover when making a loop by the rear method using two clamps on a short thread

TOPIC 8.

VARIOUS TYPES OF KNOT

Running simple knot

The running simple knot is important to learn. Its structure is based on a "false" loop (Fig. 8.1).

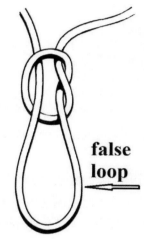

false loop

Fig. 8.1. Running simple knot

The loop is called "false" because when the free ends of the threads are pulled the loop does not tighten into a knot, but, on the contrary, one of the threads is pulled out and the whole knot is undone.

Although the running simple knot has limited use in surgery in its pure form, because it is so easily undone, it can be a part of more complex structures. In particular, the ending of a continuous suture and the first steps in creation of an Aberdeen knot are similar to a running simple knot.

How to make a running simple knot

A running simple knot is made as follows.

Thread grip. No particular thread grip is required (Fig. 8.2).

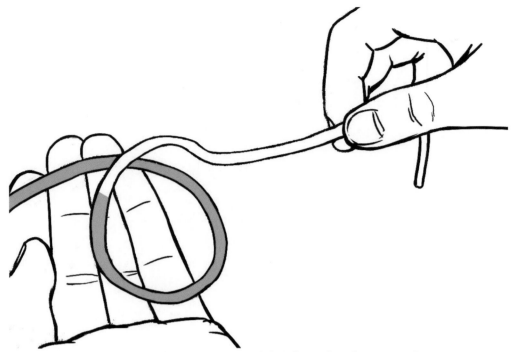

Fig. 8.2. The crossover of the thread makes a circle

Making the crossover (Fig. 8.2).

Making the false loop. The side of the thread is pushed into the ring (Fig. 8.3), creating the false loop (Fig. 8.4). The false loop is held and the ends of the thread are pulled tight to create the running simple knot (Fig. 8.5).

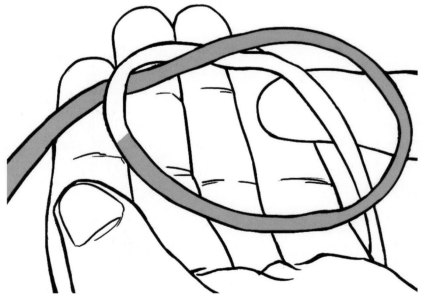

Fig. 8.3. Pushing the side of the thread into the ring

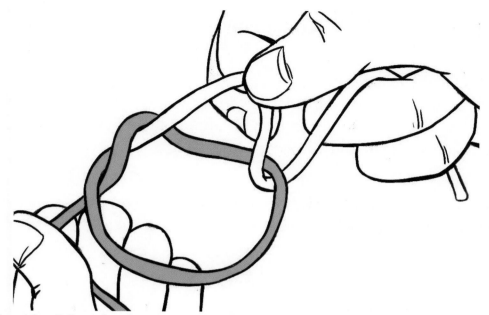

Fig. 8.4. The side of thread is driven into the ring, the ends of the thread are held in pressure grips

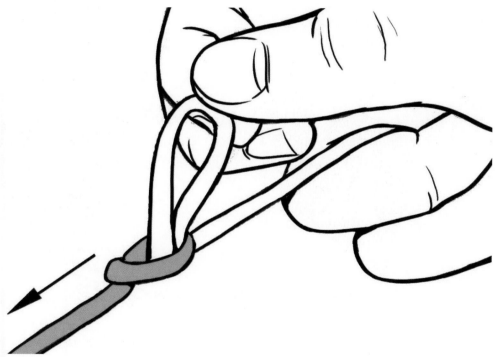

Fig. 8.5. The false loop is held by the right hand. The ends of the thread are pulled tight to make the running simple knot

The knot can be undone by releasing the false loop and pulling the ends of the thread.
Task. Make a running simple knot.

Aberdeen knot

The Aberdeen knot is made as follows.

Preparation. One end of the lace is fastened to a post on the training device and the second end is wound 3 or 4 times in a spiral around the tubes of the training device (Fig. 8.6), imitating a continuous suture.

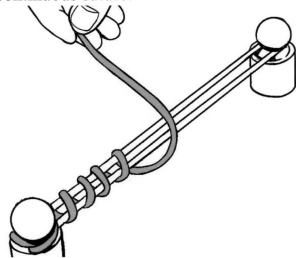

Fig. 8.6. Imitation of a continuous suture on the training device

Running simple knot. The clamp is pushed under the last spiral from the inside (Fig. 8.7), catches the thread and pulls it sideways back under the spiral to make a false loop (Fig. 8.8). The running simple knot is then tightened (Fig. 8.9).

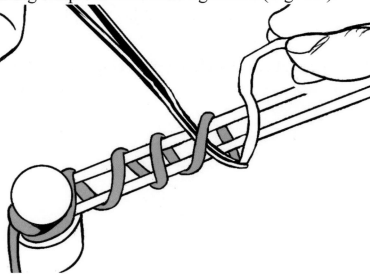

Fig. 8.7. The clamp is pushed under the last spiral from the inside and catches the free end of the thread

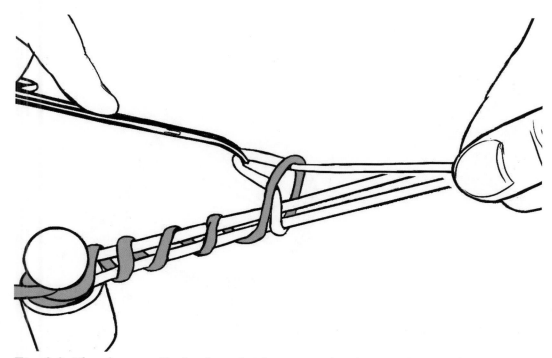

Fig. 8.8. The clamp pulls the thread sideways under the spiral to make a false loop

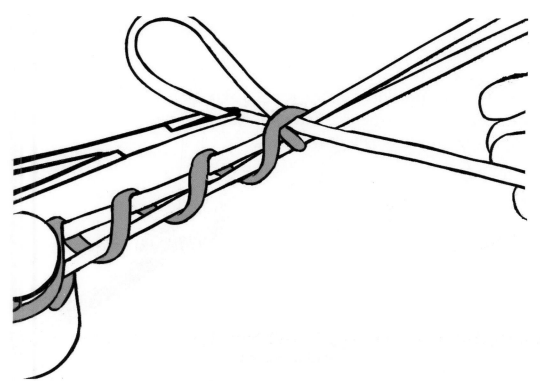

Fig. 8.9. The clamp holds the false loop, a running simple knot is made

Second false loop. The clamp is pushed through the first false loop and again catches the thread, pulling it sideways into the loop to make a second false loop (Fig. 8.10).

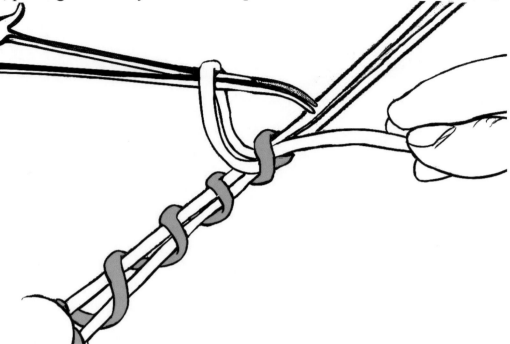

Fig. 8.10. Start of the second false loop. The clamp is pushed through the first false loop to catch the thread

Third false loop. The previous stage is repeated creating a third false loop.
Completion of the weave. The free end of the thread is pushed through the third false loop (Fig. 8.11) and the knot is tightened (Fig. 8.12).

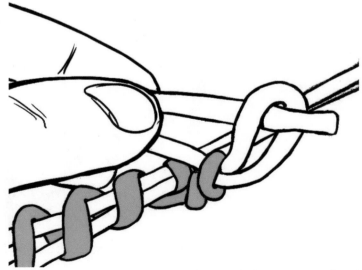

Fig. 8.11. The end of the free thread is pushed through the third false loop

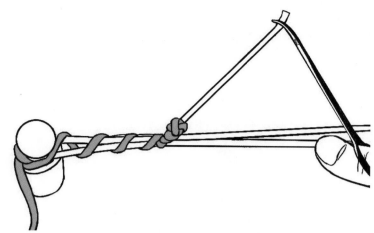

Fig. 8.12. The free end of the thread is tightened. The Aberdeen knot is made

The Aberdeen knot saves thread, marks sections of a continuous suture where it bends, and can be used to terminate a continuous suture in both open and laparoscopic operations.

Task. Make an Aberdeen knot on the training device.

Terminating a continuous suture

A continuous suture can be simply and reliably terminated by a knot made from the end of thread and the loop of the last stitch (Fig. 8.13).

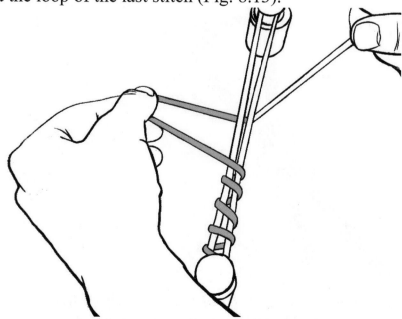

Fig. 8.13. Imitation of a continuous suture. The last spiral remains untightened

91

A continuous suture can be terminated as follows.

Preparation. Make an imitation of a continuous suture on the training device.
Making the knot. The last spiral is left untightened. The knot is made using the tip of the thread and the loop of the last stitch (Fig. 8.14).

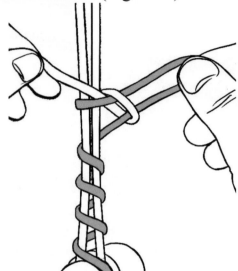

Fig. 8.14. Making a right loop with the tip of the thread and the loop of the last stitch

Task. Terminate a continuous suture on the training device.

Roeder knot

The Roeder knot and its analogues are widely used in laparoscopic surgery (Fig. 8.15). The knot is made as follows.

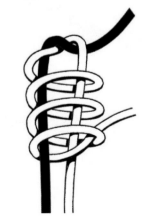

Fig. 8.15. Structure of the Roeder knot

Making a right loop. A right loop is made but not tightened on the training device. The crossover is held in place by fingers 1–2 of the left hand and the end of thread is held in a pressure grip using fingers 3–4–5 (Fig. 8.16).

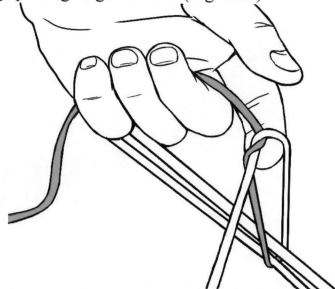

Fig. 8.16. Making the right loop. The left hand holds the thread in a pressure grip using fingers 3–4–5, the crossover lays on finger 2 before being compressed between fingers 1–2

Making a spiral. The right hand makes three spirals with the thread clockwise around the loop (Fig. 8.17).

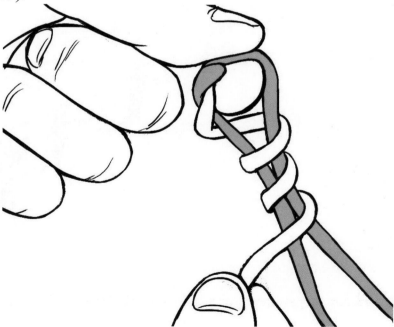

Fig. 8.17. The left hand keeps hold of the thread. The right hand makes three clockwise spirals with the thread around the untightened loop

Fixing the spiral. At the start of the fourth twist the tip of the thread is pushed through the ring of the loop and between the second and third twists of the spiral (Fig. 8.18).

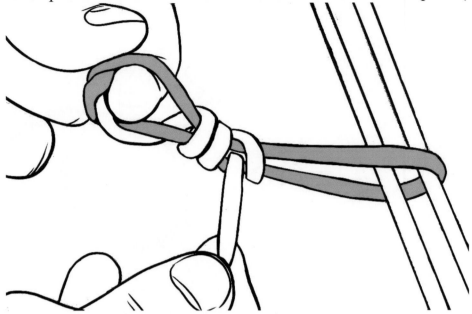

Fig. 8.18. The left hand keeps hold of the thread. The other end of the thread is pushed through the ring of the loop and between the second and third twists of the spiral

Making the knot. The Roeder knot should be properly shaped. This is achieved by uniform tensioning of all of the threads that meet in the knot (Fig. 8.19).

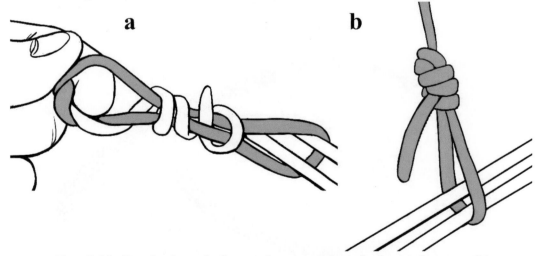

Fig. 8.19. Roeder knot before tightening (a) and after tightening (b)

Checking the loop. After the knot is tightened, it should slide along the thread quite easily, but only in one direction. The loop should remain tight when the loop ring is stretched.

Task. Make a Roeder knot.

Sliding knot

Despite appearances, the only difference between the structure of a sliding (square) knot and that of an ordinary square knot is the direction in which the threads are tightened (Fig. 8.20).

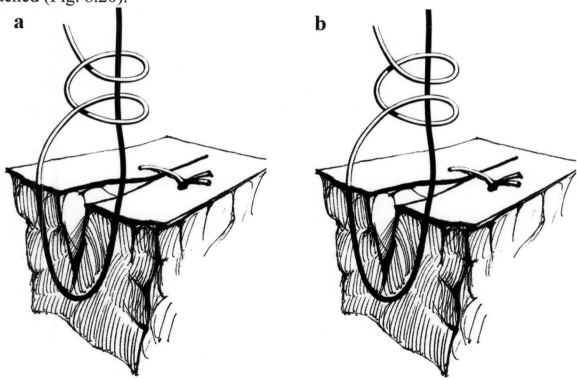

Fig. 8.20. Crossed (a) and square (b) sliding knots

A sliding knot is made as follows.

Preparation. Make a loop by the lower mirror method, holding the end of the thread in the right hand.

Thread grip. The left hand keeps the start of the thread under tension towards your body, and all the loops are tightened along it.

Making a sliding crossed knot. The right hand makes two consecutive loops (breaking the rules stated above) and this is most easily done by the lower mirror method. The loops are tightened after another along the start of the thread, which is kept taut by the left hand (Fig. 8.21). The hands do not change places (the left hand keeps hold of the start of the thread and the right hand holds the end).

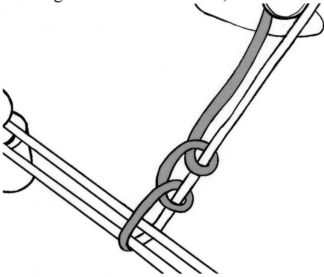

Fig. 8.21. Two loops of a sliding crossed knot, tightened along the start of the thread, kept under tension by the left hand

Making a sliding square knot. Similarly, to the sliding crossed knot, two loops are made by the lower mirror method and the hands do not change places, but different hands are used to make the right and left loops. The loops are tightened only along the start of the thread, which is kept taut by the left hand (Fig. 8.22).

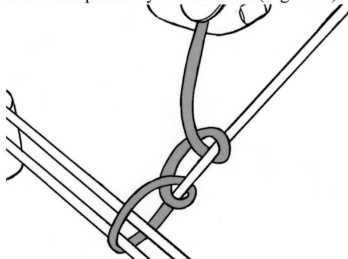

Fig. 8.22. Two loops of a sliding square knot, tightened along the start of the thread, which is kept taut by the left hand

Special features of the sliding knot. A sliding knot can be moved along the thread, tightening the loop. However, unlike a properly made Roeder knot, it can easily be undone. Sliding loops are called "asymmetrical" due to the "wrong" thread direction, and the whole sliding knot is called an "asymmetrical knot" (see Fig. 8.20).

It is important to remember that even 10 sliding loops in a knot, for example, sutures on a large artery, will not prevent an asymmetrical knot from coming undone as a result of the constant pulsation of the arteries and vibration of the suture. Depending on various factors (suture material, shape of the knot, density, diameter and pulsation force of the vessel, etc.) the knot may come undone almost immediately or after a few days. A sliding knot may be formed by incorrect tightening or twisting of threads, and by incorrect alternation of loops.

In practice a sliding knot is sometimes used in order to pull tissues together uniformly without the threat of suddenly coming undone. In this case, the sliding knot must be secured with a symmetric knot to avoid coming undone.

Task. Make a sliding square knot and a sliding crossed knot.

TEST QUESTIONS AND TASKS

8.1. Take a standard training lace (60 cm) and make several running simple knots on it, as shown in Fig. 8.23. Pull the ends of the lace in opposite directions. What happens?

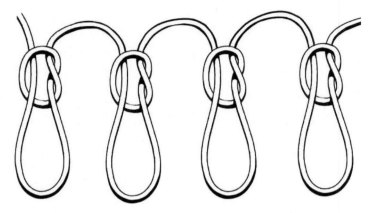

Fig. 8.23. Four running simple knots

8.2. Make an Aberdeen knot without a clamp. Then make an Aberdeen knot by the same sequence of steps, but using a clamp. Figs. 8.24, 8.25 offer guidance.

Compare classic termination of a continuous suture (using the tip of the thread and the loop of the last stitch) and termination using an Aberdeen knot as regards the amount of suture material used and the possibility of continuing the suture beyond the termination.

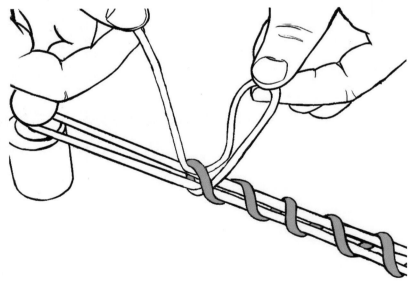

Fig. 8.24. Making the first loop of an Aberdeen knot

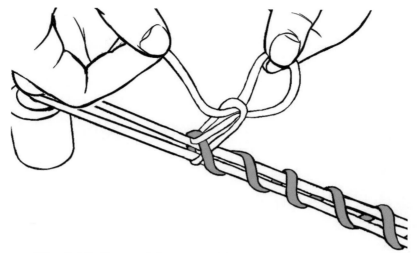

Fig. 8.25. Start of the second loop of an Aberdeen knot

8.3. Make a sliding square knot and an ordinary square knot. Compare how they resist coming undone (by stretching the loop of the knot with your hands or by inserting the clamp into the loop).

8.4. Make Roeder knots with different sorts of lace (different thickness and weave). Use two or three different types with standard length of 60 cm. Remember that it is important to ensure that the knot is properly shaped. Compare how well Roeder knots made with different laces resist coming undone.

TOPIC 9.

DIRECTION OF LOOP TIGHTENING, POSITIONING OF KNOTS

Methods and directions of loop tightening

The optimal direction for tightening of the threads when making loops depends on the shape of the loop itself and should be a natural continuation of the threads as they exit the loop. The training device provides optimal conditions for making loops, with the free ends of the thread almost perpendicular to the "wound edges" and in the same plane (Fig. 9.1).

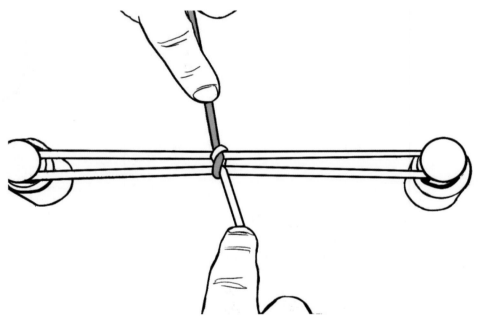

Fig. 9.1. Tightening of loops perpendicular to the wound with finger 2.

However, in practice there is not always enough room in the wound for free movement of the hands, so that an optimal position is not possible. The priority in such cases is to ensure that the exiting threads are as near as possible to being perpendicular to the wound and in the plane of the loop. This can be achieved by movement of fingers 2 only (Fig. 9.2).

100

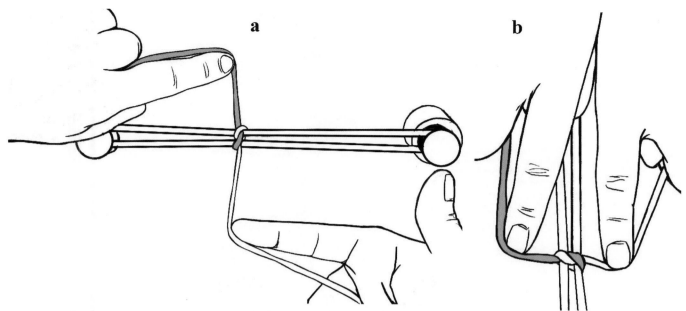

Fig. 9.2. Options for loop tightening by movement of fingers 2 only, with hands parallel to the wound: a – fingers 2 facing each other; b – fingers 2 parallel

Other methods of loop tightening may work better for some positions of the hands relative to the wound, for example, tightening with fingers 1–2 (Fig. 9.3), with fingers 1 only (Fig. 9.4), by winding the thread around finger 2 (Fig. 9.5), etc.

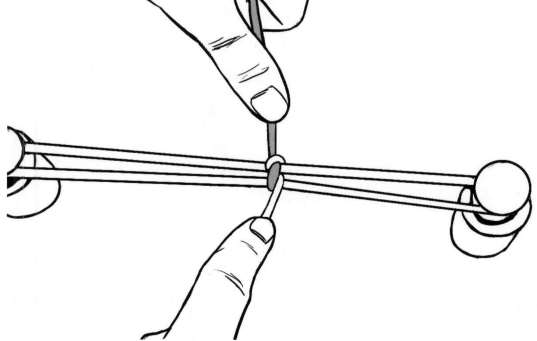

Fig. 9.3. Loop tightening with fingers 1–2

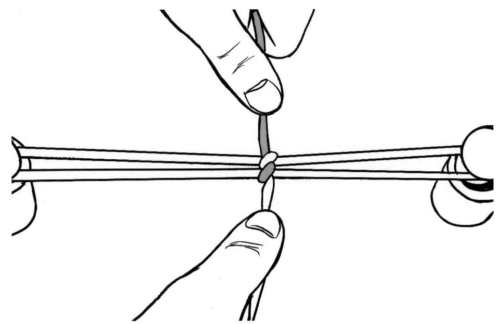

Fig. 9.4. Loop tightening with fingers 1

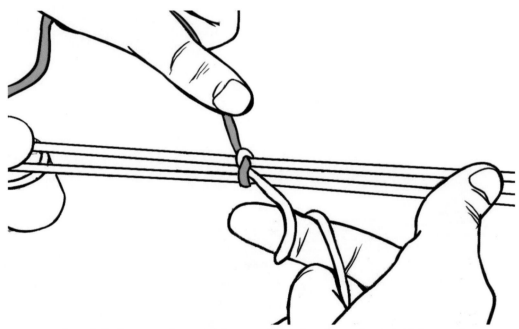

Fig. 9.5. Loop tightening by winding the thread around finger 2

These methods are not difficult to master and should be applied intuitively, as circumstances dictate.

Task. Tighten loops on the training device perpendicular to the "wound" using the methods described above.

Changing the direction of loop tightening

In practice, not only is it not always possible to tighten the loop perpendicular to the wound, but it is sometimes hard to clearly distinguish start and end of the thread. In such a case, it is permissible to tighten the loop parallel to the wound. Regardless whether it is a right or left loop, tightening with the right hand is directed to the right away from the knot, and with the left hand to the left, but the alternation of right and left loops must always be observed (Figs. 9.6, 9.7).

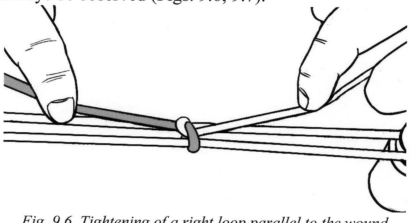

Fig. 9.6. Tightening of a right loop parallel to the wound

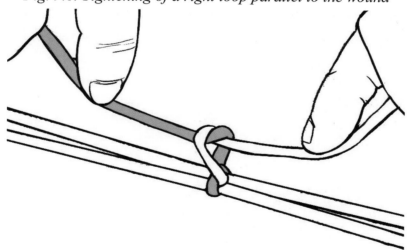

Fig. 9.7. Tightening of a left loop parallel to the wound to make a square knot

Loops should not be made in this way during routine training, because it makes it harder to establish a proper idea of loop geometry. In practice, non-standard tightening is often used in the depth of a wound, usually by experienced surgeons who are skilled at making knots in difficult conditions and without visual control.

Task. Make loops and knots, pulling the thread parallel to the edges of the wound.

Position of knots in a simple interrupted suture

When making a simple interrupted suture on the surface of the skin, the knot itself should not be located above the wound (Fig. 9.8).

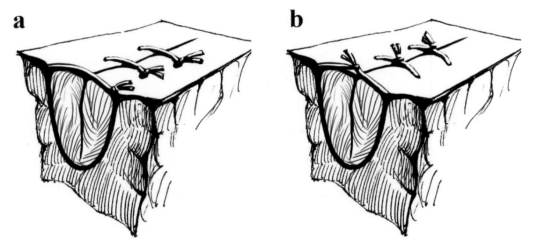

Fig. 9.8. Correct (a) and incorrect (b) positioning of the knot. The knot should not be located above the wound

All knots should be tied to one side, adjacent to one of the skin punctures (Fig. 9.9). This can be achieved by shifting the loop with the index finger (finger 2).

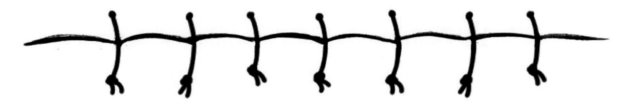

Fig. 9.9. Suture knots on the skin, correctly located to one side of the wound

Shifting a loop with the index finger

The loop has to be shifted using the index finger (finger 2) of one hand only.
Preparation. The loop has been made, but not tightened. The start of the thread is held in a pressure grip by fingers 3–4–5, while the tip of finger 2 of the same hand presses on the crossover (Fig. 9.10).

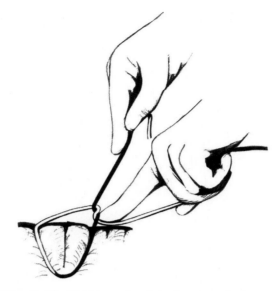

Fig. 9.10. Shifting the first loop with finger 2

Tightening the loop. The loop is tightened and shifted by tensioning of the end of the thread and unbending of finger 2 against the crossover. The end of the thread is stretched and shifts towards your body until it is almost parallel to the start of the thread (see Fig. 9.10).

Positioning of the knot away from the wound is achieved by shifting of two loops one after the other by this method (Fig. 9.11).

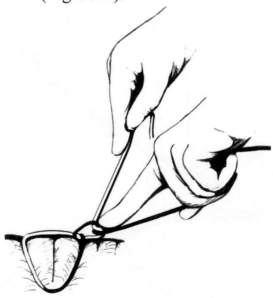

Fig. 9.11. Shifting a second loop using finger 2 to make a square knot where the thread exits from the skin

This method can be practised on the training device: the loop is shifted towards your body and tightened on the near-side tube (Fig. 9.12).

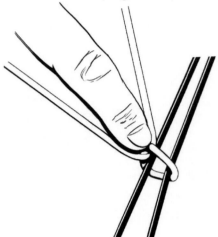

Fig. 9.12. Shifting the first loop using finger 2 on the training device

It is important, when tightening the loop, to keep the index finger pressed against the crossover and between start and end of the thread. Otherwise the loop may be deformed and become a sliding loop.

Task. Make loops by the front method with shifting of the knot.

TEST QUESTIONS AND TASKS

9.1. Making a loop on the training device by the front and rear methods. Change the position of the training device from time to time, turning it gradually (clockwise or anti-clockwise). Maintain the direction of loop tightening perpendicular to the wound in all positions of the training device (Fig. 9.13). Note how difficult it is to do this.

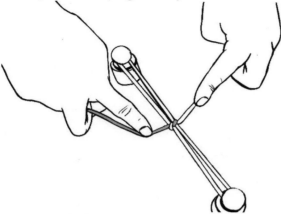

Fig. 9.13. The training device is angled, but the direction of loop tightening (perpendicular to the wound) is maintained

9.2. Use two identical laces. Compare double square knots made with tightening of loops perpendicular to and parallel to the wound.

9.3. Place the training device in a box about 15–20 cm deep, as shown in Fig. 9.14. Try making square knots on the training device when it is in the box. Which direction works best for tightening of loops – perpendicular or parallel to the wound?

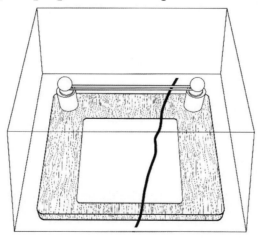

Fig. 9.14. Training device placed in a box about 15–20 cm deep

9.4. Make a square knot on the training device and try to shift the knot to the side by tightening the loop with the index finger (Fig. 9.15). Check the result.

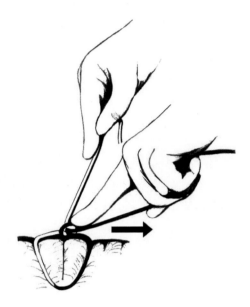

Fig. 9.15. Shifting the knot towards the skin puncture

TOPIC 10.

SECURING AND RELEASING THE THREAD WITH THE CLAMP, SECURING THE THREAD WITH THE CLAMP

If the surgeon wants the theatre nurse to pass the thread to him/her with the end of the thread held by the tip of a clamp, he/she may give the order by saying, "Thread in clamp," or "Thread on string" (length and thickness of the thread is stated separately). The tip of the clamp can hold the thread in two different ways: the end of the thread may "go into" and be entirely grasped by the tip of the clamp (Fig. 10.1); or the end of the thread may protrude from the tip of the clamp (Fig. 10.2).

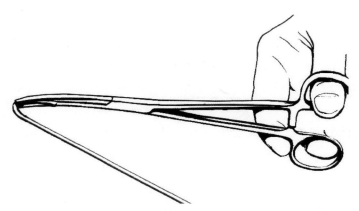

Fig. 10.1. The thread "goes into" the tip of clamp, the end of the thread is grasped by the clamp

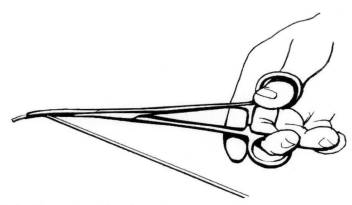

Fig. 10.2. The end of the thread protrudes from the tip of the clamp

These two threads hold must be distinguished, since they have different practical uses. The term "thread-in-clamp" is used for the first hold (see Fig. 10.1), while "thread-on-string" is used for the second (see Fig. 10.2).

Task. Grasp the thread with the clamp in two ways, as shown in Figs. 10.1, 10.2.

Thread–in–clamp

"Ligation" is the sealing of a vessel, or of a section of tissue together with a vessel, that has been compressed by a hemostatic clamp. The fragment of thread with a knot that remains on the vessel after its ligation, and which includes the ring of thread, the knot and the cut ends of the thread above the knot, is usually called a "**ligature**" (Fig. 10.3).

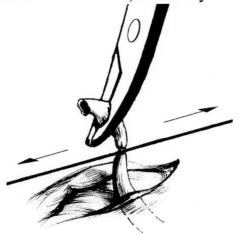

Fig. 10.3. Ligation

Thread-in-clamp can be used for ligation deep inside a wound.

Preparation. The thread is held in the clamp. The clamp is gripped in the right hand. The clamp (like surgical scissors) is always positioned in the hand with the concave side towards the midline. The clamp is held in the palm of the hand and the fingers are not fully inserted into the clamp ring.

Passing the ligature under the hook of the training device. The free end of the thread is held under tension by the left hand. The clamp is in the right hand (Fig. 10.4). A ligation can then be simulated by passing the thread around the hook of the training device. A knot is then made on the hook, with or without use of the clamp.

110

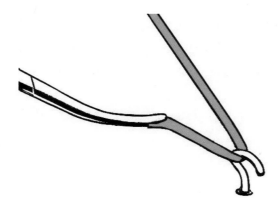

Fig. 10.4. Ligation of the hook of the training device by thread-in-clamp

Making a ligature under the thread of the training device. The thread is held by the clamp and the free end of the thread is held in a pressure grip using fingers 4–5 of the right hand, which does not prevent the same hand from holding the clamp (Fig. 10.5). The thread should be under moderate tension.

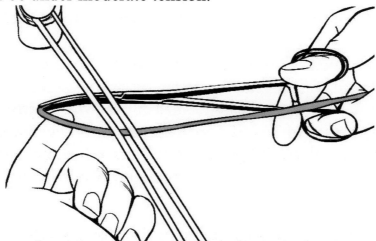

Fig. 10.5. The thread is caught by finger 2 of the left hand

Thread-in-clamp is passed under the tubes of the training device and is grasped on the other side by finger 2 or finger 3 of the left hand (see Fig. 10.5). The thread grip with fingers 4–5 is relaxed and the left hand pulls the thread under the tubes of the training device.

Alternatively, thread-in-clamp can be passed under the tubes from one side to be grasped on the other side by a second clamp (Fig. 10.6). The clamp in the right hand is then opened and the thread is pulled through.

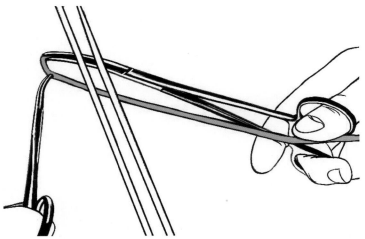

Fig. 10.6. Catching the thread with a second clamp

Task. Use thread-in-clamp to make a ligature on the hook of the training device and to pass the thread under the tubes of the device. Occasionally change the position of the training device by turning it.

Carrying the thread with a clamp

This technique is most often used for carrying the thread or an elastic holder under any anatomical structure (vessel, duct) that needs to be drawn aside. Either an ordinary hemostatic clamp or a dissector can be used. The tip of the thread should protrude from the instrument by 1–1.5 cm (Fig. 10.7). A curved clamp should be used for carrying the thread.

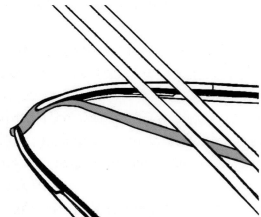

Fig. 10.7. Carrying the thread under the tubes of the training device and grasping the tip of the thread with a second clamp

When carrying the thread under the tubes of the training device it is important to keep the tip of the thread straight. Otherwise, it will be difficult to catch it with the second clamp. The way to do this is by ensuring that not too much of the thread protrudes from the first clamp.

If it proves difficult to catch the tip of the thread, the surgeon can instead catch it "by the string" (Fig. 10.8).

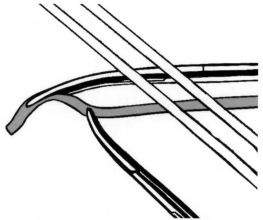

Fig. 10.8. Passing the thread and catching it with a second clamp "by the string"

It is important to remember that medical instruments require careful handling. If a good, new clamp is used to grip thick, dense threads, the instrument will soon become deformed and be incapable of holding slender threads.

Task. Carry the thread with a clamp under the tubes of the training device and catch it with a second clamp, by the tip and "by the string". Occasionally change the position of the training device relative to your body.

Removing clamp in any position

It often happens during a surgical operation that a hemostatic clamp needs to be released without changing its position. For example, if the clamp is lying on a blood vessel, a ligation has been performed, and a sudden shift of the instrument could rupture the vessel and cause bleeding. The clamp can be loosened or lifted slightly on the ratchet side (Fig. 10.9), but it must not be turned on its axis or in circular motion.

The clamp may be in any position (Fig. 10.10). In most possible positions, it will be hard to insert fingers of the right hand into the clamp rings in order to remove it. You should therefore learn to close and open the clamp without inserting fingers into the rings in the usual way, and to do so in any clamp position relative to your body, using the right and (especially) the left hand.

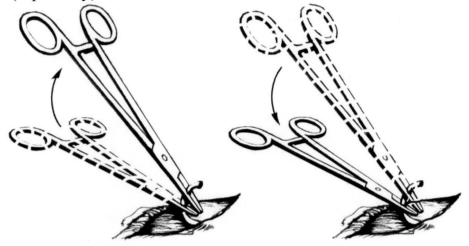

Fig. 10.9. Possible movements of the clamp in the ligation process

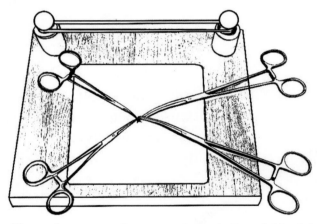

Fig. 10.10. Clamp lying on a ligature, at 2, 4, 7 and 10 o'clock positions

Preparation. Any point in the middle of the field of the training device is taken to represent a ligature held in the clamp. The clamp is placed in various positions around the ligature, with clockwise alternation.

Release and re–application of the clamp. The clamp positions change, it is released and applied again, using the right hand when the clamp rings are on the right (at 12–6 o'clock positions), and using the left hand when the clamp rings are on the left (at 6–12 o'clock positions) (Fig. 10.10).

Particular points for the left hand. It is very important to master this exercise with the left hand. The fingers should not enter the rings of clamp. One clamp ring is held by being pressed into the palm with finger 3, and fingers 4–5 are bent for extra strength (Fig. 10.11).

114

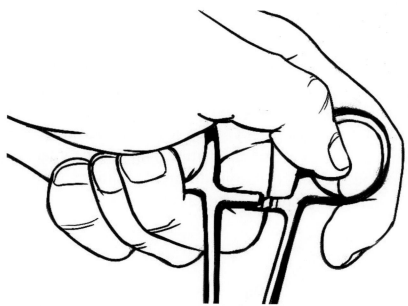

Fig. 10.11. Opening/closing the clamp with the left hand without inserting fingers into the rings

The clamp is opened and closed with finger 1 only, and the finger is not inserted into the ring, but manipulates the clamp by pushing or pulling the clamp ring (Fig. 10.11). **Particular points for the right hand**. The clamp can be closed and opened in the usual fashion with fingers 1–3, but it can be closed and opened without inserting finger 1 into the clamp ring, similarly to the way this is done in the left–hand method (Fig. 10.12).

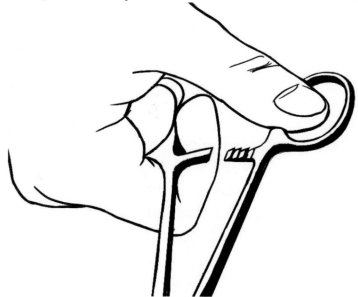

Fig. 10.12. Opening/closing the clamp with the right hand without inserting fingers into the rings

In the operating theatre, the hemostatic clamp is opened at the command of the surgeon tying the ligature. If the ligature is tightened along the edge of the clamp or where a large mass of tissue is being held, the clamp is opened slowly as the loop tightens in order to prevent the thread cutting into the tissues. If there are no tissues under tension, the clamp may be removed after the knot has been made.

The clamp must be opened more slowly when it is holding more tissues, so that the surgeon can smoothly compress the tissues with a loop of the thread.

Task. Learn to open the surgical clamp in different positions with the left and right hand without changing its position and at different speeds.

TEST QUESTIONS AND TASKS

10.1. Pass the thread under the hook of the training device using a clamp, with thread-in-clamp and the tip of the thread inside the hook. Remember that the hook of the training device is here imitating a clamp laid on a vessel in the wound. After passing the thread under the hook, decide what would be the best way of making the first loop: with a clamp (Fig. 10.13) or without.

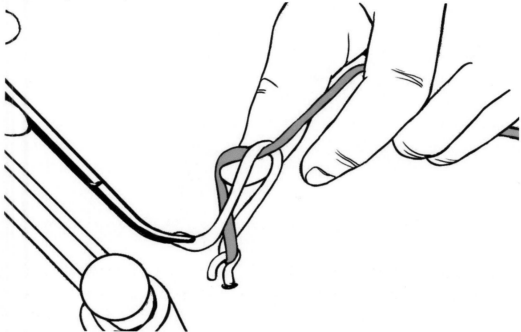

Fig. 10.13. Thread crossover when making a loop using the front method on the hook with a clamp

10.2. Why does it often happen in practice that the hemostatic clamp has to be removed with the left hand?

10.3. Opening and reapplying the clamp with right and left hands may sometimes prove difficult due to rigidity of the ratchet and overall size of the instrument. Opening the clamp may put the tissue, which it was applied to, under stress. Compare different clamps and choose the one that you find easiest to open.

Why is it important to open the clamp as smoothly as possible and without jerks?

TOPIC 11.

USE OF SCISSORS AND SCALPEL

Balancing with scissors

It is a pleasure to watch a surgical team at work when the assistant manages to make the knot and cut the thread faster than the operator turns the needle into the needle holder for the next suture. No surgeon should ever make speed an object in itself, but work that combines technical proficiency with rapidity deserves respect.

Such skillful work requires dexterity in the making of knots, but it also requires a high degree of competence in work with surgical scissors. The following exercise trains the right hand to hold the scissors in resting position with fingers 4–5 when making a knot, with quick transition to the working position in order to cut the threads. The exercise will prove much easier if you have already mastered opening and closing of the clamp with fingers 1–4.

Balancing the scissors is a matter of quick transition between the working and resting positions. In the working position the scissors are held by fingers 1–4 (Fig. 11.1).

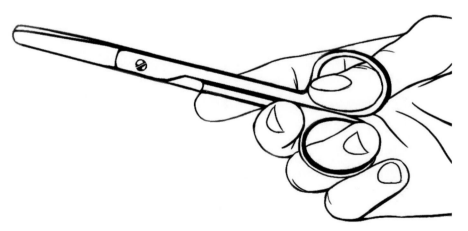

Fig. 11.1. Working position of scissors, held by fingers 1–4

In the resting position the scissors are pressed firmly against the palm of the hand by fingers 4–5 (Fig. 11.2). Finger 4 is in the ring of the scissors and finger 5 presses the other ring against the palm without being inserted into the ring.

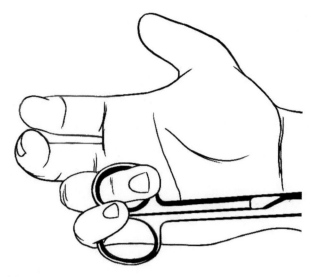

Fig. 11.2. Scissors in resting position held by fingers 4–5

It is important to note that finger 4 remains inserted into the ring of the scissors in both the working and resting positions. The scissors "spin" on finger 4 for changeover between the two positions. The concave side of the scissors should face the midline, regardless which hand they are held in.

Task. Balance the scissors on finger 4 of the right hand, alternating between the working and resting positions.

The resting position of the scissors in the right hand should not interfere with the creation of loops and knots by the left hand (Fig. 11.3).

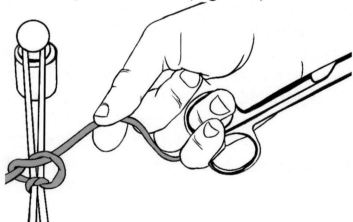

Fig. 11.3. Simultaneous thread grip by fingers 1–2, and scissor grip by fingers 4–5 of the right hand when making a loop with the left hand

Task. Make a loop with the left hand, alternating front and rear methods, while holding the thread with fingers 1–2 of the right hand and holding the scissors with fingers 4–5 of the right hand (see Fig. 11.3).

Use of scissors with the left hand

It can be hard to make cuts using the left hand, even with the best scissors, since scissors are sharpened for work with the right hand. You should remember this when making cuts with the left hand.

When you use the left hand to cut, you need to create pressure on the scissor rings in the same direction as if you were cutting with the right hand (Fig. 11.4). So, the top ring of the scissors in the left hand should be pushed away from you with finger 1, which is quite awkward to do and requires practice.

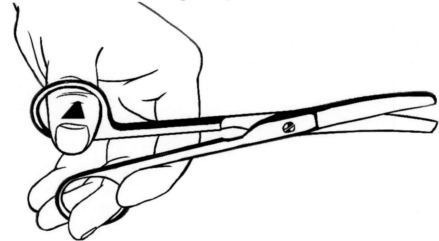

Fig. 11.4. Direction of pressure on the scissor ring with finger 1 of the left hand

You can check that scissors are sharp by using them to cut 3–4 layers of gauze. The motion should be smooth, with the threads of the gauze cut cleanly. The scissors, which you use for practice, do not need to be ultra-sharp.

Task. Take a few different pairs of scissors (some of them can be a bit loose), which cut paper and gauze well enough when held in the right hand, and learn how to cut paper and gauze holding the scissors in the left hand.

Cutting suture material with scissors

Cutting suture material with scissors above the knot is a frequent action in the course of any operation. Despite apparent simplicity of the action, there are several things that can go wrong: damage or destruction of the knot, cutting the threads too short or too long, damage to surrounding tissue, tearing of the thread, knot, loop and tissue. So, it is important to acquire proficiency.

Fig. 11.5 shows the standard design of surgical scissors.

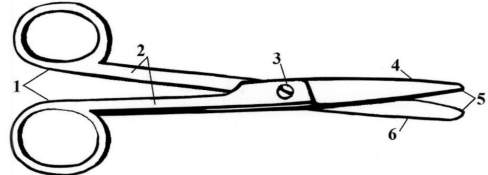

Fig. 11.5. Parts of a pair of scissors: 1 – ring; 2 – shaft; 3 – pivot; 4 – narrow blade; 5 – blade tips; 6 – wide blade

Preparation. Make a knot on the training device (on the tubes or the hook), using a piece of ordinary suture thread. The scissors are held by fingers 1–3 or fingers 1–4 of the right hand. Finger 2 of the right hand is positioned by the pivot (Fig. 11.6). The left hand holds both of the threads to be cut, applies slight tension and drives the threads apart in order to make the knot and cutting point more clearly visible.

Remember that if the scissors curve towards the tip, the curve should be towards the midline. If the scissors have one blade wider than the other, the wide blade should be below (closer to the tissue) when the scissors are in use.

Using the scissors. The scissors are brought towards the threads that are to be cut. In order to avoid any damage to surrounding tissues, the cut should always be made as close as possible to the blade tip (Fig. 11.7).

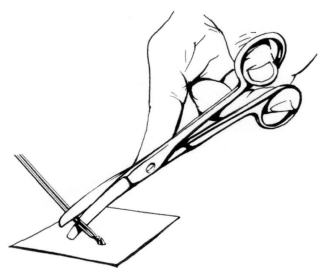

Fig. 11.6. The scissors are held by fingers 1–3 of the right hand, finger 2 is laid on the pivot, the thread to be cut is under tension and stretched away from the surgeon's body for a better view of the cutting point

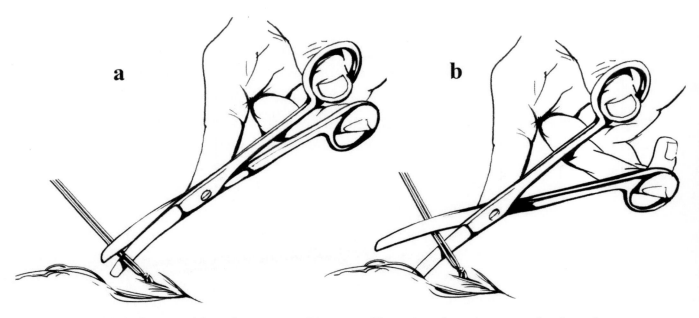

Fig. 11.7. Correct (a) and incorrect (b) ways of bringing the scissors to the threads

Hold the scissors parallel to the surface of the sutured tissues and perpendicular to the threads (Fig. 11.8) about 1–2 cm above the knot. Gauge visibility and distance from the knot to the intended cutting point (the scissors obstruct the view).

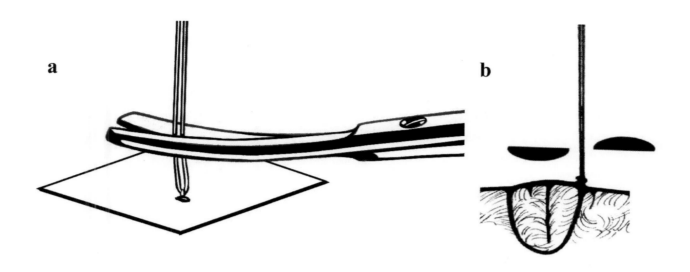

Fig. 11.8. Position of scissors parallel to the tissues (a); schematic view (b)

Cutting the thread in this position only works for surface sutures (for example, after making a suture on the aponeurosis or skin, when visibility from the side is not closed and distance from the knot to the cutting point can be gauged by sight). In such a case, it is better to use straight scissors and, if the scissors are curved, they can be held with the curve directed outwards. However, this technique should not be used in the exercises that follow, since its application is limited.

Position the scissors at an angle to the surface of the sutured tissues and threads, 1–2 cm above the knot (Fig. 11.9). Gauge visibility and distance from the knot to the intended cutting point. In this position the scissors obstruct the view less.

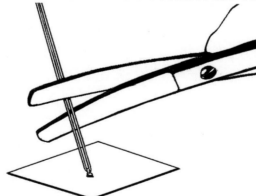

Fig. 11.9. Position of the scissors at an angle to the surface of the sutured tissues and threads

Shifting the scissors. Shift the scissors along the thread until they reach the tissue and knot (Fig. 11.10). The angle of rotation adjusts the level at which the threads are cut. The thread is kept under tension until the cut has been completed.

123

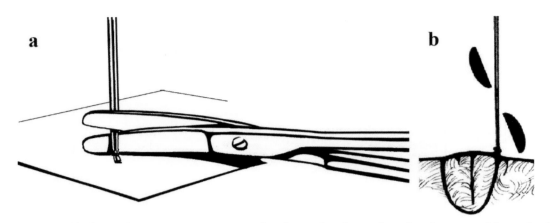

Fig. 11.10. Shifting the scissors at an angle along the thread to the tissue and knot (a, b)

Cutting the thread. When cutting the thread, always try to have a clear view of the cutting part of the scissors and of the thread between the knot and scissors (Figs. 11.7, 11.10). Make a visual check that the thread has been cut cleanly and completely.

Task. Cut the thread with the right or left hand when making sutures, positioning the scissors at an angle.

The thread ends above the knot are often called "tails" or "whiskers". Modern suture material is non-reactive, and leaving a few millimeters of tails is unproblematic (the amount of thread in the knot and loop is much greater), but you should still try not to leave too much suture material in the tissue. When doing the exercises, try to keep the tips of threads no longer than 1–2 mm long. Remember that the strength of the knot does not depend on the length of the tails.

When dense, monofilament suture material is left deep inside tissues, the tips of the threads should be cut as short as possible, since they are quite sharp. Long, sharp tips can damage surrounding tissue and even pierce adjacent structures (a duct, vessel or wall of the intestine) due to movements of the patient's organs after surgery. Such thread should be cut directly above the knot (Fig. 11.11).

Sufficiently long thread tips should be left on single sutures made on the skin.

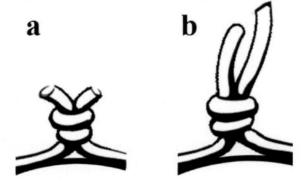

Fig. 11.11. Short (a) and long (b) thread tips above the knot

Cutting tissue with scissors

Several types of scissors are used in surgery. Dissecting scissors are mainly used for cutting and separating soft tissue. The should be used carefully, remembering that they will stop working properly if applied to tough materials (Fig. 11.12).

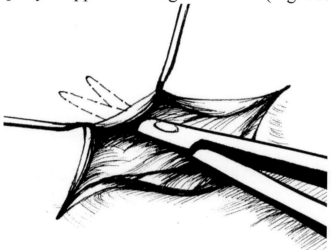

Fig. 11.12. Cutting skin with dissecting scissors

Task. Review the various types of scissors used in surgery practice. Note their length, different curvatures (along the plane and along the edge), size, width and shape of the blades, and how easy they are to handle.

Selection of a scalpel

Scalpels differ in size and configuration. Triangular, crescent and curved blades are the most commonly used. In Fig. 11.13, № 10 and № 20 are curved, № 11 is triangular and № 12 is a crescent blade.

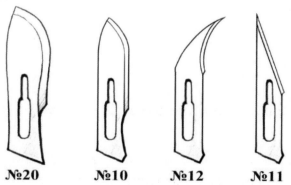

№20   №10   №12   №11

Fig. 11.13. Basic types of scalpel blade

The nature of the wound edge depends on the type of scalpel used: a sloped edge is made using a curved scalpel; a steep-edged wound is made with a triangular scalpel (Fig. 11.14).

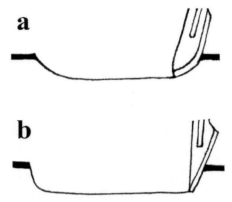

Fig. 11.14. Edges of the incision using a curved (a) and triangular (b) scalpel

The edges of the wound become mobile only where the skin is cut to the full depth, so it is best to use a triangular scalpel for small incisions (for example, to install drainage or to open a subcutaneous abscess). In long incisions and layer-by-layer dissection of tissues curved scalpels are more often used in order to reduce the risk of damage to underlying structures.

A reusable scalpel consists of a handle and a removable, disposable blade (Fig. 11.15, 11.16). The scalpel handle is attached to the blade by a special serving plate with guide slots for a hole in the scalpel blade.

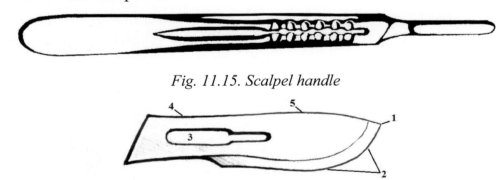

Fig. 11.15. Scalpel handle

Fig. 11.16. Scalpel blade: 1 – tip; 2 – cutting edge; 3 – mounting hole; 4 – base; 5 – spine

Task. Examine the different sort of scalpel blade that are used in surgery practice. See how their shape matches their purpose.

Attaching the blade to the handle

Important: Be extremely careful to avoid self–injury when working with a scalpel. Obtain instruction from an experienced colleague before attempting to assemble or disassemble a reusable scalpel. Injury can result from failure to follow the correct procedure, excess effort (not required when the procedure is properly followed) and haste.

Assembling the scalpel. The scalpel blade is best held by the spine with a hemostatic clamp or needle holder (Fig. 11.17a). The mounting hole must remain open. The clamp with the blade is held in the right hand. The plate on the scalpel handle fits into the mounting hole on the blade (Fig. 11.17b). The blade moves along the guide slots on the plate until its base clicks into place (Fig. 11.17c). The scalpel is now fully assembled.

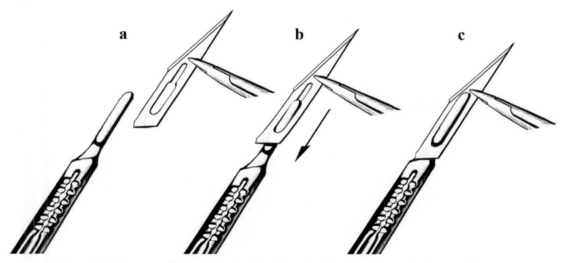

Fig. 11.17. Assembling the scalpel (a–c). See the description in the text

Disassembling the scalpel. The scalpel is held with the cutting edge away from the body (Fig. 11.18a). The blade is held with a clamp or needle holder at the base and pulled above the plate of the handle (Fig. 11.18b). The blade is shifted off the plate (Fig. 11.18c). The scalpel is now fully disassembled.

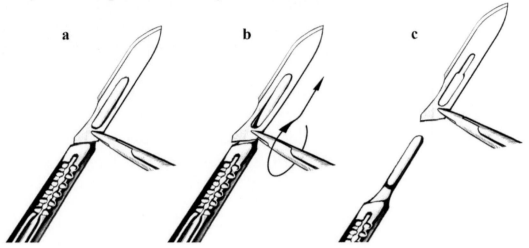

Fig. 11.18. Disassembling the scalpel (a–c). See the description in the text

Making an incision with a scalpel

The basic positions of the scalpel in the hand are: the pencil grip, bow grip and knife grip (Fig. 11.19–11.21). The ball and trocar grips are also used. The choice of grip depends on the scalpel blade, its handle and the practical task to be carried out.

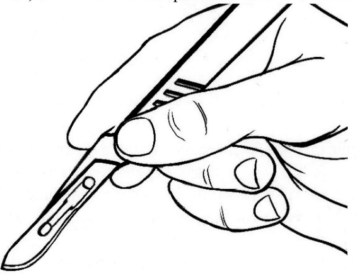

Fig. 11.19. Scalpel in the pencil grip

The pencil grip is optimal for small incisions (with a triangular scalpel, or with a curved scalpel if there is a risk of damage to underlying structures). The bow and knife grips are mainly used with curved scalpels when making long incisions, when finger 2 can rest on the scalpel blade in a supporting position.

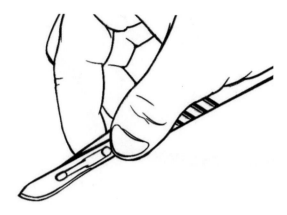

Fig. 11.20. Scalpel in the bow grip

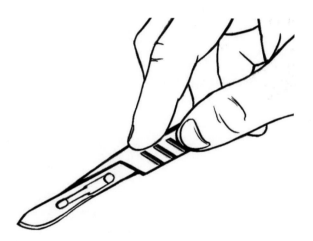

Fig. 11.21. Scalpel in the knife grip

Notice that the pencil, bow and knife grips allow smooth change in the angle between scalpel and skin along the incision, which is important because the scalpel normally assumes a near vertical position at the start and end of the incision. The angle of inclination is reduced along the main part of the incision and depends particularly on the type of blade. The optimal angle can be felt depending on how easily the tissue is dissected. You should always aim to cut the tissue in layers.

Task. Alternate between the basic scalpel grips in the dominant hand.

Skin incision with a triangular scalpel

A skin incision with a triangular scalpel is made as follows.

Preparation. Mark the incision line on the tissue with a pen or marker and decide on the required depth of the incision (for example, 2 cm). Take a disposable triangular scalpel in the right hand in the pencil or knife grip (Fig. 11.22).

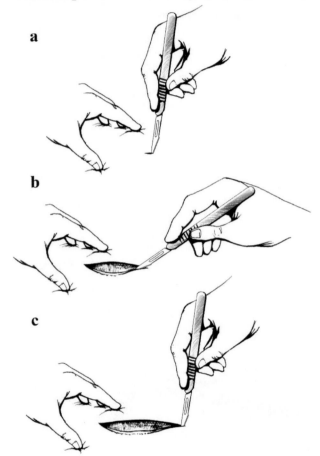

Fig. 11.22. Making an incision with a scalpel (a–c). See the description in the text

Before the start of incision, the skin is pressed with the left hand and slightly stretched away from the incision to prevent excessive movement (Fig. 11.22a).

Puncturing the skin. The scalpel is positioned vertically with the tip on the point where the incision will start. The tissue is punctured to the desired incision depth (Fig. 11.22, a).

Execution and completion of the incision. The scalpel tilts to an angle of 30–40 degrees and the incision is made along the previously drawn line (Fig. 11.22b). At the end of the incision line the scalpel is brought to almost vertical position, making the wound edge almost vertical, and is withdrawn (Fig. 11.22c).

Practise making incisions on artificial materials and also on natural materials (such as pork shin) and try making incisions with various scalpel types.

Task. Make a tissue incision using a triangular scalpel.

TEST QUESTIONS AND TASKS

11.1. Assess the grip of scissors in the hand, shown in Fig. 11.23. What is wrong with it?

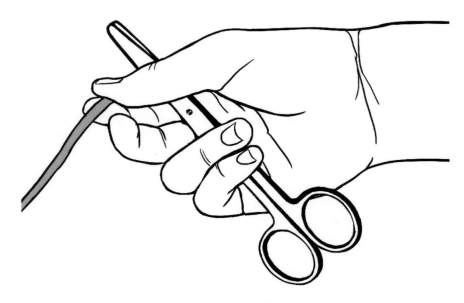

Fig. 11.23. Scissors held in fingers 4–5

11.2. Which scalpel blade (curved or triangular) is better suited for long incisions and which is better suited for short incisions?

11.3. If the tips of the thread above the knot were accidentally cut too long (for example, 15-20 mm instead of 2-3 mm), should they be left as they are or shortened. If they are to be shortened, what is the best way to do it? Try shortening the length of the "tails" using scissors with the thread tips held in a clamp (Fig. 11.24).

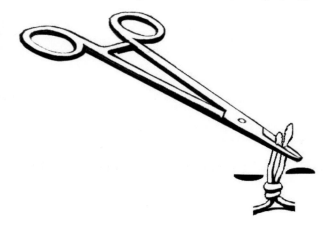

Fig. 11.24. Shortening of threads above the knot using clamp and scissors

11.4. Name the parts of a scalpel blade.

11.5. Which figure shows the optimal position of scissors and thread in order to cut the thread above the knot (Fig. 11.25a–c).

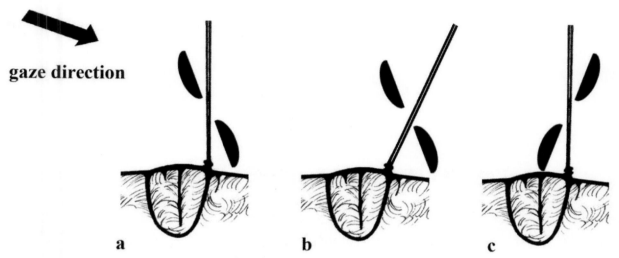

Fig. 11.25. Possible positions of scissors for cutting the thread above the knot (a–c)

TOPIC 12.

SUTURE MATERIAL

Exercises on the training device with various types of suture material are important because they give the student a feeling of how different types of needle and thread behave in surgery practice.

There are a great number of different trade names for suture materials, but the range of threads and needle types commonly used in surgery is actually quite limited.

Packaging of suture material

All manufacturers use the same system of labelling and it is important to be well versed in the terminology. As well as the brand name, packaging should have printed information on it containing chemical composition, diameter and length of the thread, size, shape and structure of the needle, shelf life, sterilization type, lot number and various other parameters (Fig. 12.1).

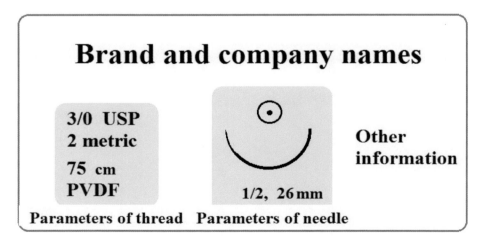

Fig. 12.1. Basic labelling of a package of suture material

Brand and company names are important for recognizability of the suture material.
Parameters of the thread:

- thread diameter (UPS size and metric size);
- thread length (for example, 30 to 150 cm);
- chemical composition of the thread (polyglycolide, polydioxanone, polyamide, polyurethane, polypropylene, polyester, polyvinylidene fluoride (PVDF, fluoropolymer), polyethylene, silk, catgut, steel;
- thread colour (white, colourless, blue, green, etc.);
- thread structure (monofilament or braid, may be indicated by a symbol);
- absorption of the thread (time required for absorption, period of tissue retention (indicated less frequently));
- breakage force (some suture materials are specially made so the thread detaches from the needle at a certain level of force; such suture material is specially marked).

Needle parameters:
- configuration of the needle tip (piercing, cutting, blunt);
- cross–section of the needle body (round, triangular (with inner or outer cutting edge), trapezoid);
- number of needles (no needle, one needle, two needles on the tips of one thread, several needles and threads in one pack);
- needle with looped thread (both ends of one thread are fixed in the eye of the needle);
- needle curvature (1/2, 3/8, 5/8) or shape of the needle;
- needle length with an image of the needle (or needles) to actual scale.

Other information:
- shelf life, storage temperature, batch number;
- "CE" labelling indicates that the materials have a certificate of compliance with the requirements of the European Union Directive on medical goods;
- warnings on packaging, often in the form of symbols (not to be reused, not to be sterilized, not to be used if the package is damaged).

Composition and properties of threads

If you know what a thread is made of, you also know whether or not it will be absorbed in the body.

Absorbable thread: polyglycolide, polydioxanone, catgut.

Partially absorbable thread (absorption takes several years): polyamide, polyurethane, silk.

Non-absorbable thread: polypropylene, polyester, polyvinylidene fluoride (fluoropolymer), polyethylene, steel, titanium.

Threads used for training are usually made from polyglycolide and polyamide.

Thread made from natural materials (silk and catgut) is no longer used in most countries due to high risk of complications. Steel and titanium are the only "natural" materials still used for surgical thread, but they have very few applications. So modern suture material is mainly synthetic.

It is obviously of great importance to know how long it takes for threads to be absorbed and how long they continue to hold tissue together. The tissue retention period is hardly ever stated on packaging. It depends on the composition and thickness of the thread, and also on the nature of the tissues to which the suture is applied. The tissue retention period is defined as the number of days for which the thread maintains >30% of its original resistance to breakage.

It is important to pay careful attention to the properties of suture material, which you are working with for the first time. Always check and double check the manufacturer's detailed description of the material.

Polyglycolide suture material may have a tissue retention period of 7 to 30 days and is absorbed within 40 to 120 days.

If the tissue retention period of polyglycolide is only 7 to 10 days, the trade name of the suture material usually includes the words "rapid" or "fast". Such material is also sometimes called "artificial catgut", and the thread is often without colouration.

Polydioxanone suture material has a tissue retention period of up to 50 days.

Absorbable thread is broken down by hydrolysis, so polyglycolide and polydioxanone thread that is kept unused beyond its shelf life can break in the body sooner than it is meant to, due to gradual hydrolytic breakdown which began in the packaging

Task. Interpret the information about thread parameters that is given on suture material packaging. Identify differences and similarities in the way the information is presented on packaging by different manufacturers.

Thread structure

The structure of surgical thread is of two main types (Fig. 12.2):

- **monofilament** (consists of a single fiber);
- **polyfilament** (consists of several fibers).

Simple twisted and braided polyfilament threads are hardly ever used in surgery today (see Fig. 12.2).

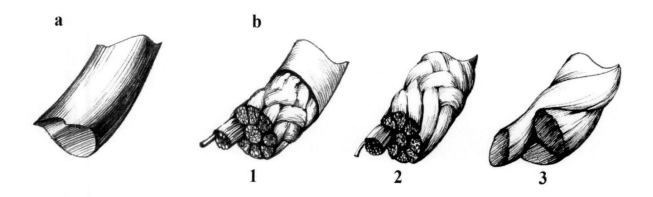

Fig. 12.2. Structure of suture materials: a – monofilament thread; b – polyfilament thread: 1 – braid with polymer coating; 2 – braid; 3 – twisted

Modern polyfilament thread is also braided, but it has either an outer polymer coating that reduces friction or is braided from fibers with different chemical structure. Such threads could be classified as multi-component, combined or complex, but they are still described as "braided".

Note that polyglycolide and polyamide thread may be braided or mono–filament. Braided polyglycolide thread usually has a polymer surface coating to reduce friction and slow down absorption. Presence of a coating will be marked on the packaging as an extra component of the thread.

Monofilament thread has a smoother surface than polyfilament thread. Less surface friction means less damage to tissues (Fig. 12.3).

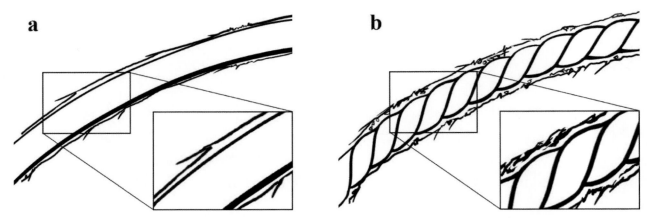

Fig. 12.3. Damage to tissue from monofilament (a) and braided (b) threads

The degree of friction can be roughly gauged by slightly compressing the thread between fingers 1–2 and pulling it with the other hand. You will feel a notable difference between monofilament and braided threads.

Diameter of the thread also has significant impact on its handling properties, which include strength, elasticity, flexibility, resilience, friction and torque.

Be aware that excessive rubbing together of the thread when making loops can lead to their rupture. The risk is greatest when tightening the second loop.

In practice, thread behaves quite differently when handled dry and when it has been wetted and covered with biological material, held in a gloved hand. Compare thread friction when dry and after being dipped in water – it will, of course, be much less in the second case. Thread can be moistened in a sodium chloride solution before use in order to lessen friction.

The thread may curl after it has been taken out of the packaging due to "shape memory". This is typical of most surgical suture materials. Some manufacturers use specially designed packaging, which automatically straightens the thread as it is pulled out of the package.

Task. Compare the handling properties of various suture materials. Compare degrees of friction when dry and wet.

Thread diameter

Thread diameter is not constant along its length, but varies within acceptable limits, so, if the metric system is used, it is necessary to specify an interval, for example the interval from 0.2 to 0.249 mm. But to spell out such intervals in full would be too long-winded for communication in the operating theatre and on packaging.

Thread diameter is usually stated on packaging by two classification systems: USP and metric size. So, for example, 3/0 in USP classification (often written "3–0" and read as "three zero") corresponds to the interval from 0.200 to 0.249 mm. In the metric description this is written in abbreviated form as "2" (Table 12.1).

Table 12.1. Diameter, labelling and use of various synthetic threads

USP	Metric size	Diameter, mm	Possible use
<6/0	<0.7	<0.070	Ophthalmology and microsurgery
6/0	0.7	0.070–0.099	Vascular surgery, liver duct system
5/0	1	0.100–0.149	
4/0	1.5	0.150–0.199	
3/0	2	0.200–0.249	Gastrointestinal tract
2/0	3	0.300–0.339	Skin, aponeurosis
0	3.5	0.350–0.399	Aponeurosis of the white line of the abdomen
1	4	0.400–0.499	

But systems (USP and metric) are normally used on packaging, but USP is most usual in oral communication.

Number of loops in a knot

More loops in a knot do not always add to its strength. Increase of the number of loops above four has very little effect on properties of the knot.

However, this is only true if all the loops in the knot are made by the same method. If, for example, the knot begins with two sliding loops, but is completed as a classic square knot, then the completion will determine the strength of the knot as a whole.

The decision how many loops to include in the knot should be based on the thickness and structure of the thread.

Suture material with USP thickness of 2, 1, 0, 2/0, 3/0 requires three loops in the knot for braided thread and four loops for monofilament thread. If the tissue is under tension, then four loops are needed for braided thread and five for monofilament. When using USP 4/0, 5/0, 6/0 thread the usual rule is: make as many loops as there are zeros in the labelling.

Mistakes in knot formation and their correction.

If you believe that you have made a mistake when tying a knot, you must inform the team, and make sure that the knot and suture are visually or mechanically solid. If you judge that the knot could be unreliable (for example, that it may slide due to twisting of the thread), you should decide the best course of action depending on the circumstances (whether the knot has already been tightened, or the thread has been cut). You can try to pull the knot tight, make an additional suture at the same place, strengthen an unreliable knot with a square knot, increase the number of loops, remove and remake the suture, or find some other solution.

Surgical needles

Structure of the needle

The needle consists of a point, tip, body and eye, and an internal and external surface (Fig. 12.4).

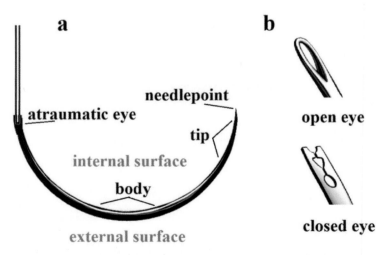

Fig. 12.4. Structure of a surgical needle (a) and its eye (b)

140

The thread is attached to the needle at the eye. Needles with open and closed eyes, which can be rethreaded many times, are rarely used because they damage the tissue (the cross section of the eye is significantly larger than the cross section of the needle body).

A needle with an atraumatic eye (an eye with diameter comparable to that of the needle body) is called an atraumatic needle. The eye of an atraumatic needle consists of a channel cut into the needle, in which the thread is gripped.

Atraumatic needles do less damage to tissue, but they cannot be threaded more than once. Reusable needles are deployed nowadays only to complete a suture after accidental detachment of an atraumatic needle, but in this case, they are not reused, but are disposed of together with the damaged atraumatic needle. However, even though reusable needles are no longer a part of standard surgical practice, they are suitable for student practice and it is worth learning how to use them.

Task. Compare the width of the atraumatic and open eye on atraumatic and reusable needles of similar size.

Labelling of needles

The label on suture packaging will show the structure of the needle, with diagrammatic cross-sections of the tip and body of the needle (Fig. 12.5).

The tip and body may have a round cross-section or may have facets. The most common needle types are round-piercing, round with a cutting tip, and reverse-cutting needles.

A round-piercing needle causes minimal damage to the tissue because it has a circular cross-section without edges along its entire length. A round needle with cutting tip has a triangular cutting tip, but its body is round in section.

A reverse cutting needle is often simply called a "cutting needle". It has a triangular cross section with cutting sides/facets along the entire length of the tip and body.

There are many variants of needle design with respective package labelling. Their names are themselves an accurate description of their structure, but a review of their properties is still worthwhile.

141

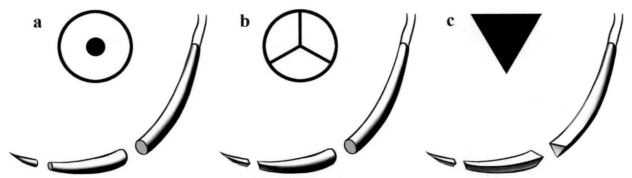

Fig. 12.5. Structure and labelling of needles: a – round-piercing; b – round with cutting tip; c – reverse cutting

Task. Study the different types of needle used in surgical practice. Match the labelling with the structure of the needle.

Curvature and shape of the needle

The curvature of the needle can be written as a fraction, which treats its length as a part of the circumference of a circle. The most common variants are 1/2 and 3/8 (Fig. 12.6), meaning that the needle's length is, respectively, a half and three-eighths of the circumference of a circle. A needle with 5/8 curvature can be used in urology for suturing of the bladder walls. Other shapes (less commonly used) are the ski, straight and J-type needles (Fig. 12.7).

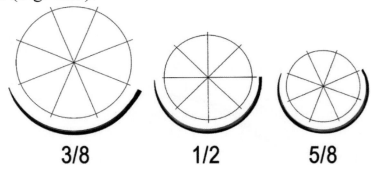

3/8   **1/2**   **5/8**

Fig. 12.6. Needle shape as part of a circle

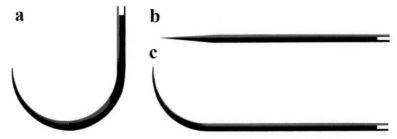

Fig. 12.7. J-type (a), straight (b) and ski (c) needles

Practice with atraumatic needles is necessary because they are what is most commonly used in the operating theatre. Any type of thread (0, 2/0 or 3/0) on needles 25 to 35 mm in size will serve for the exercises described here. The needles should preferably be 1/2 size and round, since they will do less damage to the materials on the training device.

Opening the packet, taking out the suture material

Producers of medical goods increasingly supply their materials (disposable cloths, catheters, probes, etc.) pre–sterilized, and it is important to remove them from the packaging correctly.

Materials usually come double-packed (with internal and external packaging). The outer surface of the outer packaging is non-sterile. It has all necessary information (including how long the materials will remain sterile) printed on it. This information should be read and noted. Be sure to check the outer packaging for integrity. If it is damaged, the contents cannot be used.

The outer packaging, usually consists of two sheets, one of which is paper. At the edge of the package, there will be a point where these sheets can be grasped separately. Pull them apart using two hands to gain access to the inner packaging, which is then removed with sterile forceps or a sterile hand (Fig. 12.8).

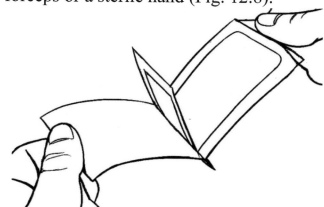

Fig. 12.8. Opening the outer suture material packaging

The outer packaging should not be opened by mechanical tearing.

Be sure to follow safety procedures after opening of the suture material packaging. Grasp the needle with a needle holder (not with hands) in order to avoid possible injury, make the training device ready for work in advance and take special care when working.

After grasping the needle with the needle holder, pull the thread out of the package (Fig. 12.9). The thread may form knots as it is taken from the packaging if it was not properly packed or if it is taken out too quickly.

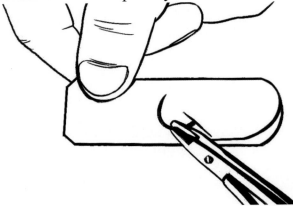

Fig. 12.9. Using a needle holder to take the needle out of the package

There is no need to dispose of the needle immediately after using the thread. Needles are quite long-lasting and for some exercises (not for making knots, but pulling threads through tissue) a needle with a short thread will suffice. Be careful how you store and dispose of needles, and always keep them in a special container.

Task. Practise proper opening of packages containing suture materials. Prepare a container for storing needles.

TEST QUESTIONS AND TASKS

12.1. Compare different suture materials by their levels of friction.

12.2. Which of the following suture materials is absorbable: polyglycolide, polydioxanone, polyamide, polyurethane, polypropylene, polyester, polyvinylidene fluoride, polyethylene?

12.3. Describe the structure of the needle based on its labelling (Fig. 12.10).

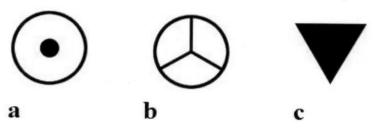

a   b   c

Fig. 12.10. Labelling of needles (a–c)

12.4. Which needles, those with curvature of 3/8 or of 1/2 (Fig. 12.11), do you think are most often made as cutting needles and which as piercing needles? Why?

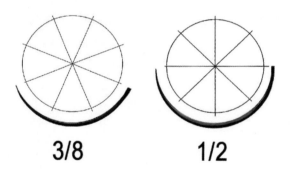

3/8   1/2

Fig. 12.11. Needle curvature

TOPIC 13.

USING A NEEDLE HOLDER AND FORCEPS

How to grip the needle holder

The optimal grip of the needle holder depends on the state of the wound, the surgeon's experience, the size of the instrument, the thickness of the needle, the density of the tissue to be sutured, and other parameters.

It is often recommended to grip the needle holder with fingers 1–3 or 1–4 (Fig. 13.1, 13.2), which is similar to grips on the clamp and other instruments.

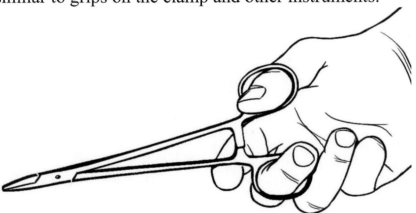

Fig. 13.1. Grip of needle holder with fingers 1–3 (supported by finger 2)

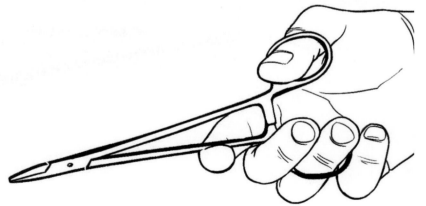

Fig. 13.2. Grip of needle holder with fingers 1–4 (supported by fingers 2–3)

The grip with fingers 1–4 (supported by fingers 2–3) gives firm command of the instrument. However, it also limits freedom of hand movement to some extent. The same applies to the grip with fingers 1–3.

Holding the needle holder in the palm of the hand (Fig. 13.3) allows greater freedom of movement and makes movement smoother. It also enables the surgeon to feel the action of the needle and tissue better. One disadvantages of this method is that it may require additional movement of the fingers in the ring in order to open the needle holder. However, a high-quality needle holder can be opened without inserting the into the ring.

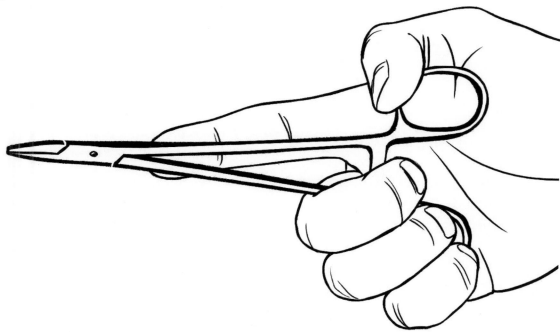

Fig. 13.3. Grip of needle holder in the palm of the hand

Overall, although holding the needle holder in the palm has some advantages, it requires special training, since it can lead to shifting of the needle when the instrument is opened.

Task. Try out the various ways of holding needle holders, reach you own opinion on the ergonomics of the various methods.

Position of the needle in the needle holder

The inner surface of the jaws of the needle holder, like those of a hemostatic clamp, are usually serrated to ensure a good grip of the needle.

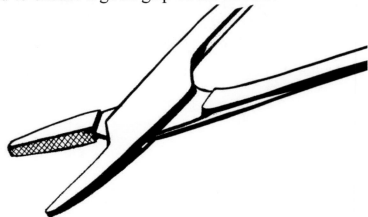

Fig. 13.4. Serrated inner surface of the needle-holder jaws

The needle is best held at a distance between 1/3 (Fig. 13.5, a) and 1/2 (Fig. 13.5, b) of the length of the needle measured from the eye, depending on the density and thickness of the tissues to be sewn with the needle. The thinner the needle and the denser the tissues, the farther from the eye and closer to the middle the needle should be held. The needle can be held for suturing from right to left and from left to right.

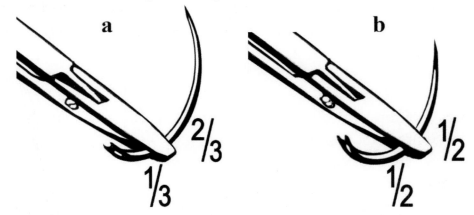

Fig. 13.5. Needle grip for suturing from right to left. See the description in the text.

The needle should be gripped as close as possible to the tip of the needle holder. Gripping the needle at the base of the jaws may damage the needle holder.

Fixing the needle in the needle holder

After removing the needle from its packaging, hold it by the tip with bent fingers 1–2 of the left hand (Fig. 13.6). Put the needle holder on the straightened finger 3 and grip the needle. This technique ensures that the needle can be fixed safely, accurately and confidently, which is especially important with small needles.

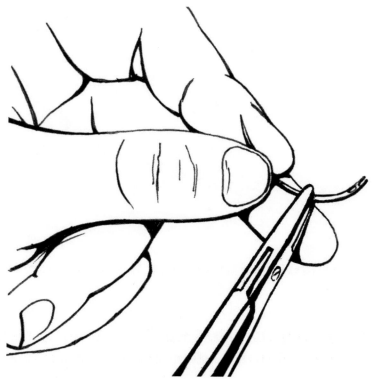

Fig. 13.6. Fixing the needle in the needle holder for a right-to-left suture

Be careful: a poor-quality needle holder may open accidentally, releasing the needle in an unpredictable direction, and scattering biological material. It is important to wear protective glasses for this reason. Accidental opening of the holder may occur if the needle has been fixed incorrectly (too close to the tip), or if the holder is defective or old, or when the needle is very thick, or if the needle is not firmly gripped (only one click of the ratchet).

Task. Fix the needle in the needle holder.

Attaching thread to a needle with an open eye

Thread is attached to a needle with an open eye as follows.

Preparation. The needle is fixed in the needle holder for a right-to-left suture. The right hand holds the needle holder (in the palm) and one end of the thread (in a pressure grip with fingers 1–2 or 3–4–5). The other end of the thread is in the left hand (Fig. 13.7).

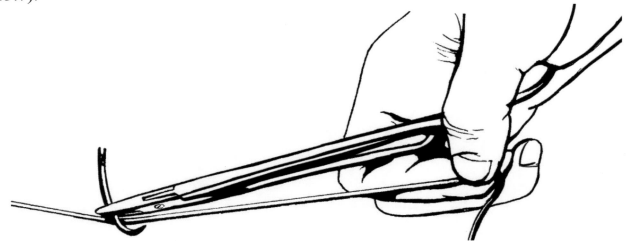

Fig. 13.7. Preparing to fix the thread in an open-eye needle

Directing the thread. The left hand stretches the thread slightly and pulls it downwards into the corner between the needle and needle holder (Fig. 13.7). The thread is then brought over the jaws of the needle holder and directed onto the eye of the needle (Fig. 13.8).

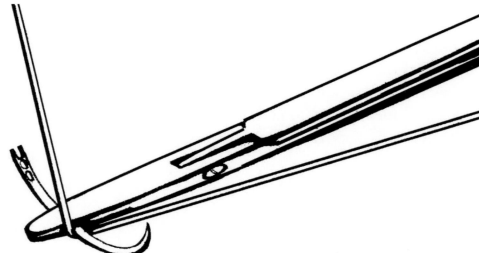

Fig. 13.8. Directing the thread into the corner between the needle and needle holder

150

Latching the thread. The thread is stretched more firmly and latched into the eye of the needle in a downward movement (Fig. 13.9).

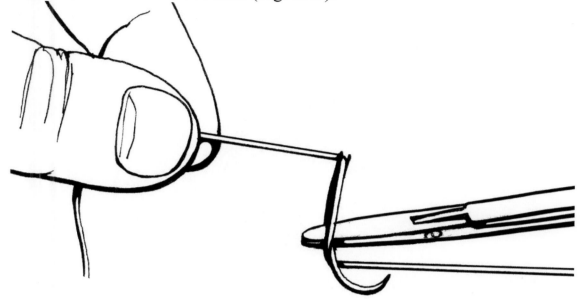

Fig. 13.9. Latching the thread in the eye of needle

Take care to avoid hurting the left hand with the needle point: ensure that the thread to be latched into the needle is long enough for the left hand to remain at a safe distance from the needle.

Task. Fix a thread into an open-eye needle.

Turning the needle in the needle holder

The needle has to be turned 180 degrees in the needle holder. There are many ways of doing this, and in practice you can choose between them depending on the circumstances and on what is most convenient.

In all of these actions, it is important to be aware of the potential danger posed by biological material during manipulations with surgical needles and instruments.

The needle is turned in the needle holder with the aid of the forceps. Use forceps that hold the needle firmly. Use the most common position of the needle in the needle holder: 1/3 from the needle eye to the point and close to the tip of the jaws of the needle holder.

Preparation. The needle is gripped in the needle holder, which is held by fingers 1–4 or 1–3 of the right hand. The forceps are held by fingers 1–2 of the left hand. Both instruments are perpendicular to a line between the surgeon's elbows and parallel to each other (Fig. 13.10).

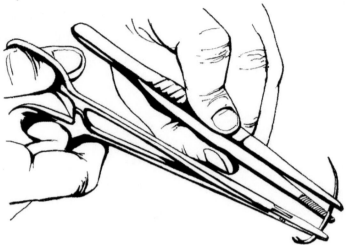

Fig. 13.10. Grip of needle with forceps, forceps and needle holder are parallel to each other

The following two methods of turning a needle in the needle holder can be used.

Method 1. Without changing the positions of the forceps and the needle holder, the needle is grasped by the forceps and immediately released from the needle holder. The needle can be grasped nearer the eye or nearer the tip, depending which way it was initially facing (see Fig. 13.10).

There are two variants for method 1:

Variant 1. Turning the needle in the forceps. The forceps are turned towards your body. The needle is also turned by 180 degrees so that its outer side is uppermost. The needle is then caught again by the needle holder without changing the position of the needle holder (Fig. 13.11);

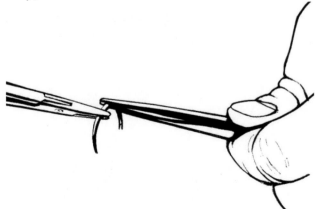

Fig. 13.11. Forceps with the needle towards your body, the needle holder again grips the needle

Variant 2. Turning the needle in the needle holder. The forceps and needle holder are turned at an angle of 90 degrees to each other. The needle holder is placed onto the forceps proximal to the needle (Fig. 13.12). The needle is gripped gently by the forceps and turned with the side of the needle holder. The needle is again fixed in the needle holder.

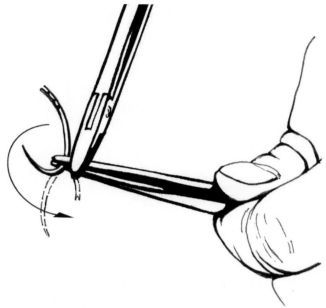

Fig. 13.12. The forceps hold the needle, which is to be turned (and already has been shifted a little in the desired direction) by the side surface of the needle holder

Method 2. The forceps turn 90 degrees to the right and grasp the needle (Fig. 13.13) which is immediately released by the needle holder. The needle can be grasped nearer the eye or nearer the tip, depending which way it was initially facing.

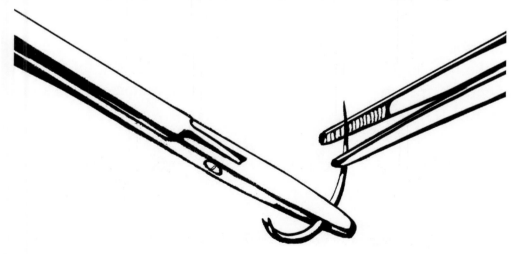

Fig. 13.13. Grip of needle with forceps, forceps and needle holder are perpendicular to each other

There are two variants of method 2:

Variant 1. Turning the needle with the forceps. The left hand is rapidly pronated, turning the forceps and needle. The needle holder grasps the needle again, without changing its position (the technique is similar to variant 1 of method 1, see Fig. 13.11);

Variant 2. Turning the needle around with the needle holder. The needle is held by the forceps and turned, being pushed by the needle holder, for example, at the needle eye (Fig. 13.14). The needle is grasped again by the needle holder, but from the other side.

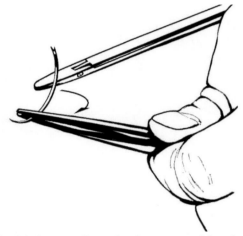

Fig. 13.14. The forceps hold the needle, which is turned by the tip of the needle holder

Task. Turn the needle in the needle holder with the forceps and needle holder using the various different methods.

Use of forceps

In surgery, the forceps are routinely used to hold or move tissues aside, and for holding and turning the needle. There are many types of forceps. They differ in size and in structure of the tip. It is important to be able to differentiate anatomical and surgical forceps (Fig. 13.15).

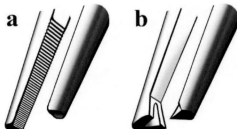

Fig. 13.15. Structure of the tips of anatomical (a) and surgical (b) forceps

Forceps can be held with fingers 1–3, supported by finger 2 (Fig. 13.16) or with fingers 1–2 (Fig. 13.17).

The forceps used for training should hold the needle firmly and not be so rigid as to strain the hand during work. Surgical forceps with large serrations will damage the surface of the training device, so it is better to use anatomical forceps when possible.

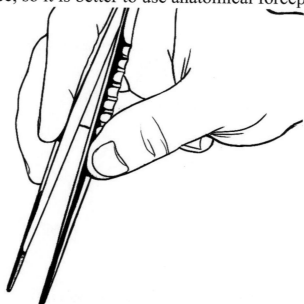

Fig. 13.16. Grip of forceps with fingers 1–3, supported by finger 2.

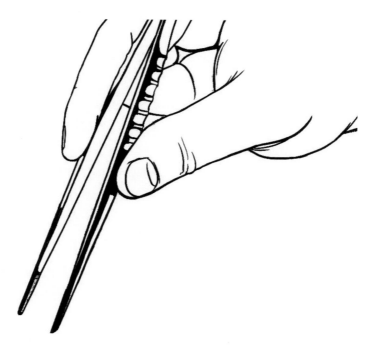

Fig. 13.17. Grip of forceps with fingers 1–2.

Task. Gauge the ergonomics and functionality of different forceps using the two different grips.

Use of forceps when making a suture

When making a dermal suture, it is not usually necessary to grips the wound edge with forceps. Piercing atraumatic needles can pierce the skin without any need to grip the wound edges. One jaw of the forceps can be used to lift the edge of the wound slightly, which will reduce damage to tissues (Fig. 13.18).

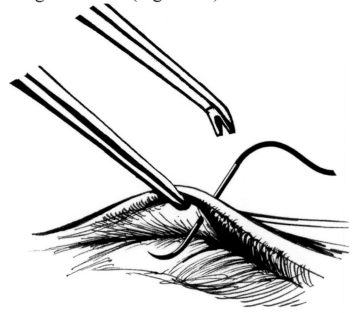

Fig. 13.18. Lifting the edge of the skin with one forceps jaw

Gripping the skin edges with forceps during suturing is not a mistake, but, in practice, it should only be done if a firm grip is absolutely essential, since unnecessary mechanical force may damage the tissues.

The main applications of the forceps during suturing are for turning the needle, temporary securing of the needle in tissues, and drawing the wound edges together.

Use of forceps in adaptation of wound edges

When making a simple interrupted suture, the wound edges may turn outwards or inwards due to reduced elasticity of the tissues or roughness of the wound edges. If this has happened, it must be corrected, because bringing together of non-matching tissues or opening of the wound cavity will impair healing.

Such turning inwards or outwards can be prevented by aligning the wound edges with forceps and holding them in position until tightening of first loop of the simple interrupted suture (Fig. 13.19).

Proper joining of wound edges in these cases can also be achieved by firm tightening of the first loop in the interrupted suture and altering the suturing method, for example, by using a vertical mattress suture.

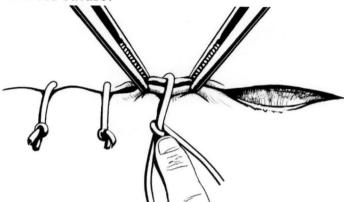

Fig. 13.19. Securing the skin edges with two forceps when tightening the first loop of a simple interrupted suture

Task. Ensure that the wound edges meet properly when making sutures.

TEST QUESTIONS AND TASKS

13.1. Name the main ways of gripping a needle holder. Work out which method you prefer.

13.2. State the rules for securing the needle in the needle holder. Which part of the needle should be longer in Fig. 13.20, part (a) or part (b)?

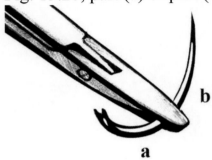

Fig. 13.20. Securing the needle in the needle holder: parts of the needle (a and b)

13.3. Decide which way of turning the needle in the needle holder works best for you. What makes you choose one way of doing it rather another?

TOPIC 14.

VARIOUS TYPES OF SUTURE

Adaptation of wound-edge rules

Extensibility and contractility of the skin in any anatomical region depends on direction, reflecting the Langer lines. In practice, this means that the shape of a wound can change greatly, immediately after it has been made. The wound edges of one and the same wound contract differently and almost always differ in length. In a complex wound, the joining together of the wound edges requires care and observance of certain rules.

Rules for joining of the wound edges. The surgical procedure should include careful examination of the opposite edges of the wound in order to identify matching damage and continuation of the natural folds. Matching damage marks on opposite sides of the wound should be located, like pieces of a jigsaw puzzle, and taken into account when making the suture (Fig. 14.1).

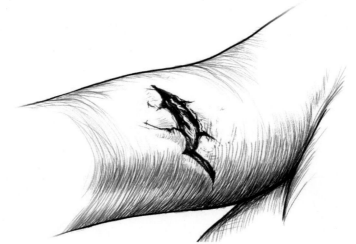

Fig. 14.1. Similar damage on opposite edges of a wound

The rule of dividing the wound in half. The lengths of the two edges of the wound are bound to be unequal, so it is recommended to make each suture by dividing the not sutured part (parts) of the wound in half. This ensures that the sides of the wound are joined at the right places (Fig. 14.2).

Task. Find matching injuries on opposite sides of the wound in Fig. 14.1.

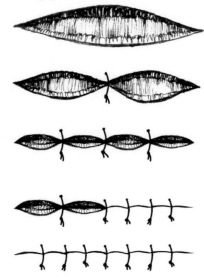

Fig. 14.2. Matching the wound edges by dividing the wound in half

Simple interrupted suture on the skin

The aim of a skin suture is accurate joining of the wound edges with minimal tension, compression and traumatization of tissues. The wound edges should be sutured in accordance with specific recommendations on the surgeon's stance relative to the wound, the choice of suture material, use of forceps and needle holder, path of the needle, and making of the knot (Fig. 14.3).

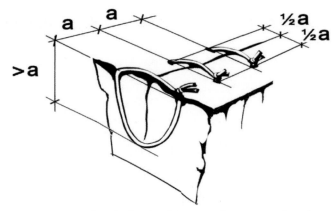

Fig. 14.3. The ratio between suture depth (>a), distance between the skin punctures in one suture (1/2a + 1/2a) and the gap between adjacent simple interrupted sutures (a)

General recommendations. The suturing depth should be deeper than the distance between the skin punctures. The gap between two sutures should be roughly equal to the distance between the skin punctures within one suture. The suture should bring the wound edges together without deformation or over-tension. The wound should be sutured in such a way that no cavity is left in the depth of the wound after the making of the knot. The knot should be located where the thread exits from the skin, and not above the wound.

Stance of the surgeon relative to the wound. You should stand so that the wound edges are parallel to a straight line between your elbows.

Task. State the rules for skin suturing using simple interrupted suture.

Removal of a simple interrupted suture

When a suture is made, the needle creates the wound channel as soon as it is applied and part of the thread remains in this channel until the suture removal. One part of the thread is inside the tissue, and the other part is outside (with the knot). Although the outer part is treated with antiseptic during dressings, it should be understood that it is no longer sterile at the time of suture removal. So, the outer, non-sterile part of the thread must not pass into the wound channel during suture removal. The in-tissue part of the thread must always be pulled out slightly (Fig. 14.4a, b) and the suture is then cut on the part that has been pulled out (Fig. 14.4c). This principle applies to the removal of any type of suture.

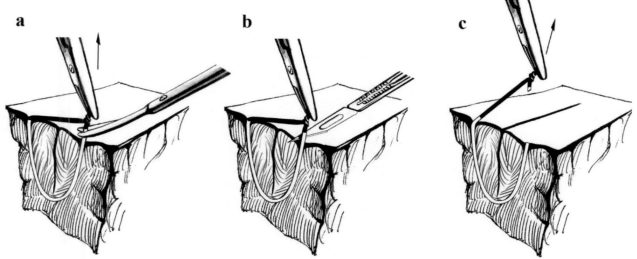

Fig. 14.4. Steps and methods for removal of a simple interrupted suture (a–c). The description is given in the text

A suture is removed using scissors as follows

Preparation. Take pointed scissors (with one or both blades sharpened) and forceps.
Pulling the suture. Grip the suture knot or tails with the forceps and pull them upwards to reveal a section of the concealed thread. If the scissors have only one sharp blade, this blade should be inserted under the thread section that has been pulled out of the tissue (see Fig. 14.4a).
Cutting the thread. The thread is cut, and the suture is pulled out (Fig. 14.4c). Inspect the suture to make sure that it has been completely removed.
Take care not to cut both threads below the knot (this is a common mistake).

A suture is removed using a scalpel as follows

Preparation. Take triangular scalpel and forceps.
Pulling the suture. Grip the knot or tails with the forceps and pull them upwards to reveal a section of the concealed thread. Insert the tip of the scalpel blade under the section of concealed thread that has been pulled out, with the scalpel spine to the skin and cutting edge facing onto the thread (see Fig. 14.4, b).
Cutting the thread. The thread is cut, and the suture is pulled out (Fig. 14.4c). Inspect the suture to make sure that it has been completely removed.
Be especially careful when working with a scalpel. It may be necessary to use a scalpel for removal of a suture if the suture is particularly small or if the suture is set deep into tissues.
Task. Remove sutures using scissors and scalpel.

Path of the needle in tissue

The needle should puncture the skin at an angle of 90 degrees to the surface of the skin (Fig. 14.5).

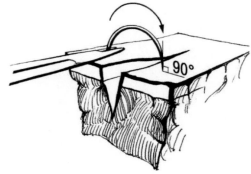

Fig. 14.5. Angle of skin puncture and trajectory of needle motion

Passing through tissue, the needle should follow a trajectory that coincides with its curvature. If the needle is shaped as part of the circumference (the arc) of a circle, it should move through the tissue along an arc with the radius of that circle.

The skin punctures should be at roughly the same distance from the wound edges. When practicing on the training device, make marks with a felt-tip pen at one-centimeter intervals along a line 0.5 cm from the wound edges (Fig. 14.6). This will help you to get the habit of a regular distance from wound edges to punctures and between punctures along the wound.

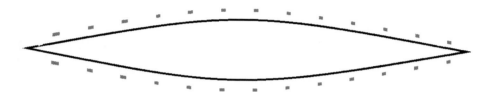

Fig. 14.6. Labelling of puncture points on the training device

Task. Mark points for punctures along the wound edges on the training device.

Vertical mattress suture (Donati suture)

The vertical mattress suture (Donati suture) enables joining of the wound edges with less tension and greater accuracy than a simple interrupted suture. This assists healing and leaves a lighter scar. Donati stitching is sometimes also called "cosmetic", although its use in mainstream surgery has become routine.

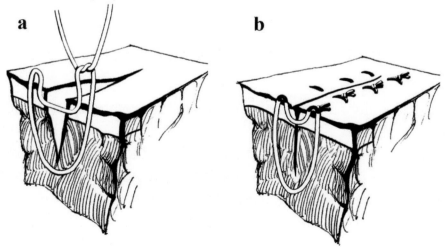

Fig. 14.7. Structure (a) and appearance (b) of a Donati suture

163

A Donati suture with an atraumatic needle requires two stitches in the wound edges, passing in opposite directions.

Step one: stitching the dermis. First, only the edges of the skin are sutured. The puncture is made at 3-5 mm from the wound edges to a depth of 1-2 mm without piercing right through the dermis. The opposite edge of the wound is sewn in the same way but in reverse order (Fig. 14.8).

Step two: stitching the skin. The thread is pulled through after suturing of the dermis, and the needle is turned 180 degrees. The left hand grips both ends of the thread exiting from the skin and uses them to pull up the wound edges (Fig. 14.9). The next punctures are made no less than 10 mm away from the wound edges, stitching the skin in the opposite direction. The thread is pulled through and the knot is made.

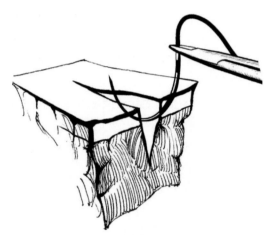

Fig. 14.8. Step one of a Donati suture (stitching the dermis edges)

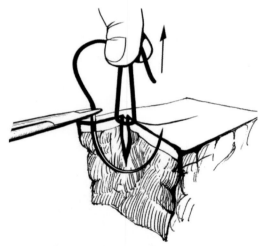

Fig. 14.9. Step two of a Donati suture (stitching the skin)

The two steps of the Donati suture can be reversed (the skin is stitched first and then the dermis), and this is usually done when large volumes of tissue need to be joined and the wound edges cannot be drawn together with a single movement of the needle, or when the needle is not long enough for this.

Task. Practise the Donati suture on the training device.

Removing a Donati suture

After a Donati suture has been made the knot is on one side of the wound and a small section of thread (part of the loop) that needs to be removed is on the other side. Forceps or a hemostatic clamp are used to catch the small section of thread and pull it upwards until the tread emerges from the skin at the two adjacent punctures. The emerging thread is cut with scissors just above each of the punctures (Fig. 14.10).

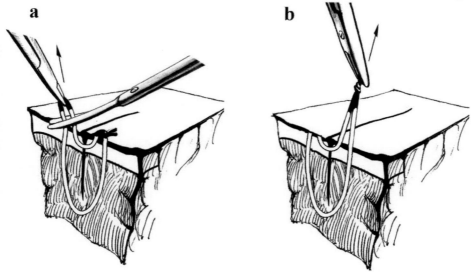

Fig. 14.10. Removal of a Donati suture: cutting (a) and removal (b) of the thread

If it is hard to grip the section of loop on the skin, a Donati suture can be removed in the same way as a simple interrupted suture.

Task. Remove a Donati suture on the training device.

Fixation of a drainage tube to a stitch

A drainage tubes can be conveniently held in place by attaching it to a nearby single stitch on the wound.

Tubes 25-30 cm long from an infusion system can be used as drainage tubes for practise purposes. The arrangement can be simulated on the training device by making two parallel incisions on the fabric of the training device, each about 2 cm long, at a distance of 4-5 cm from each other. The tube is pulled under the fabric of the device from one incision to the other so that its ends protrude from the incisions (Fig. 14.11).

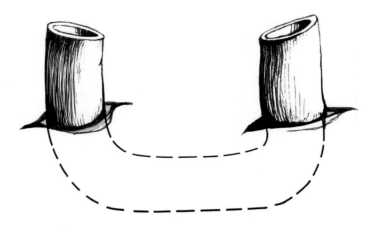

Fig. 14.11. Modelling of wounds with a drainage tube on the training device

The tube can be tied to an adjacent simple interrupted stitch (or a Donati stitch), by running threads around it from two sides and tying a knot (Fig. 14.12a). In some cases, a "bridle" is created between the suture knot and the drainage tube (Fig. 14.12b), by the insertion of an extra knot. Such a bridle gives the drainage tube a certain mobility and makes it easier to remove the drainage tube while leaving the suture in place Always draw both threads around the drainage tube, going right around the tube with both threads (not just one), in order to hold the tube firmly in place.

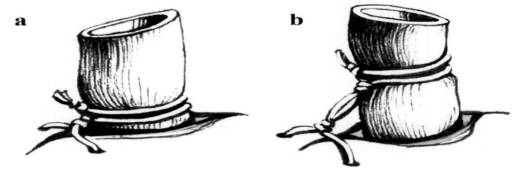

Fig. 14.12. Fixing drainage tubes to simple interrupted sutures with both threads going right around the drainage tube: a – without bridle; b – with bridle

Several steps are required to fix a tube on the training device with a bridle.
Preparation. Make a simple interrupted suture next to the tube. A bridle 1.5-2 cm long is created by making a second knot on the thread (Fig. 14.12b).
Passing the threads around the tube. The key to passing the threads around the drainage tube is the transfer from hand to hand, which should be done quickly and almost without looking at the hands.

There are several ways of transferring the threads from hand to hand. It is most easily done in front of the tube (Fig. 14.13). Use the same actions as for making a loop by the rear mirror method and for one-step creation of complex loops (these manipulations include transfer of the threads from hand to hand).

The actions required for transfer of the threads behind the drainage tube are shown in Figs. 14.14, 14.15.

The holding knot. After the holding knot has been made, the thread should slightly compress the drainage tube (see Fig. 14.12a, b), but without excessive narrowing of its inner passage. Make sure that the tube is firmly secured.

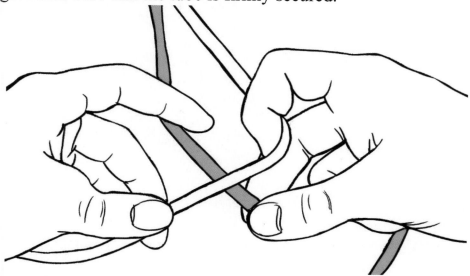

Fig. 14.13. Transferring the threads in front of the drainage tube with fingers 2, from prior grip with fingers 1–3

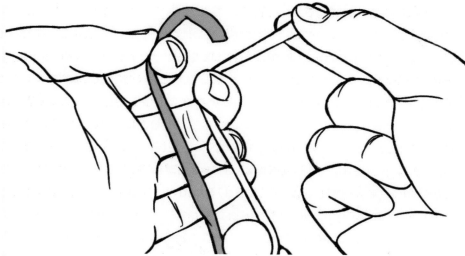

Fig. 14.14. Starting transfer of the threads behind the drainage tube from initial grip with fingers 1–2

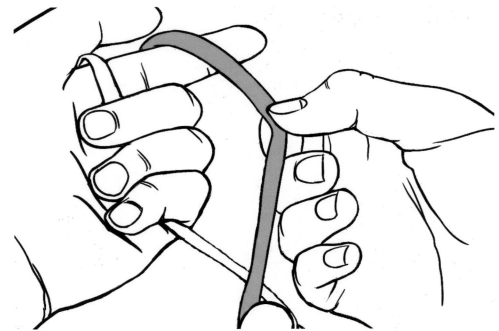

Fig. 14.15. Completion of transfer of the threads behind the drainage tube from initial grip with fingers 1–2

Tasks. 1. Practise transfer of the threads from hand to hand behind and in front of the drainage tube. Pay attention to the initial thread grip and be clear about the order of the main actions.

2. Fix a drainage tube on the training device with and without a bridle.

Continuous intradermal suture

Removable continuous intradermal sutures are widely used in surgery. They are usually defined as cosmetic (Fig. 14.16).

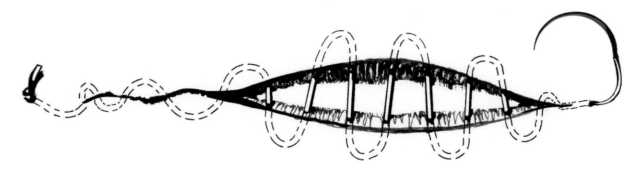

Fig. 14.16. Continuous intradermal suture

A continuous intradermal suture is carried out as follows.

Start of suture. The first stitch is made at the level of the dermis only. It begins with a skin puncture at 8–10 mm from the corner of the wound, driving the needle through the dermis towards the corner of the wound (Fig. 14.17).

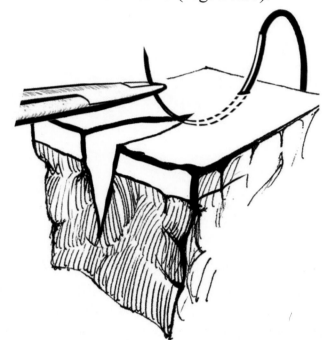

Fig. 14.17. Start of an intradermal suture, suturing the corner of the wound

First stitch. The first stitch must begin from the corner of the wound, otherwise the edges of the dermis at the corner will not come together. All the stitches should be of the same depth, without piercing right through the dermis or epidermis (they should remain in the dermis layer) and should gather the same volume of tissue.

Alternate edges of the wound are then stitched in a chessboard pattern. The exit of the needle from the dermis on one side of the wound should be opposite the place of entry of the needle into the dermis on the other side of the wound (see Fig. 14.16).

Intradermal continuous suture with a loop. If the intradermal suture is long, there is a risk that the thread will break when it is being removed, making it hard to extract the remainder of the thread. This problem can be avoided by stitching one loop of the suture outside the skin when the suture is made (Fig. 14.18). The needle is punctured through the skin to the outside, then re-enters the skin on the opposite side of the wound and comes out of the dermis on the side of the wound to continue the intradermal suture.

Clips or knots can be applied on the ends of the threads to anchor them on the skin. Knots on the thread ends are made by the wind-around method using a needle holder right on the surface of the skin (for example, the double academic knot, $+2-2+2$, may be used). The knot should be strong (although there is almost no load on it) and of large size to prevent it from slipping under the skin. It is important to calculate properly where the knot at the other end of the thread is to be located (the best location depends on the tension of the wound edges).

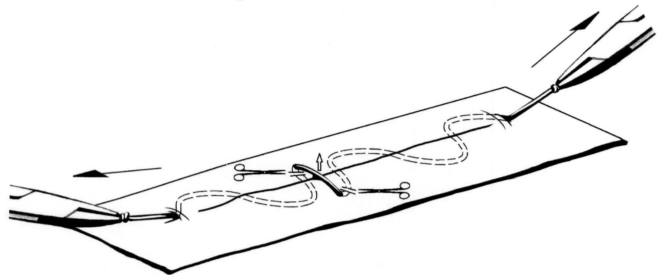

Fig. 14.18. Removing the loop and entire suture of a continuous intradermal suture

Removal of an intradermal continuous suture

If a loop above the skin was made as part of the suture, removal of the suture is the same as for the Donati suture. The loop is pulled up so that a part of the thread emerges from the skin, and the emerged part of the thread is cut with scissors on both sides (see Fig. 14.18). The thread is pulled out by the end knots.

If there is no loop in the suture, one of the knots is pulled up, the emerged thread is cut (Fig. 14.19a) and the thread is pulled out by the second knot (Fig. 14.19b).

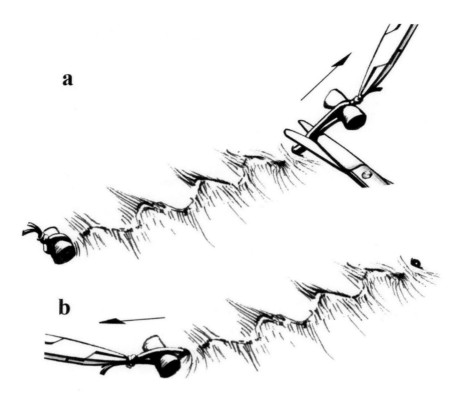

Fig. 14.19. Stages in removal of an intradermal continuous suture (a, b). The description is given in the text

Task. Make a knot at the end of the thread on the training device by the wind-around method using a needle holder.

Purse–string, Semi-purse-string and Z-shaped sutures

The purse-string, semi-purse-string and Z-shaped sutures are commonly used in surgery. Their structure is made clear by the illustrations below (Figs. 14.20, 14.21, 14.22).

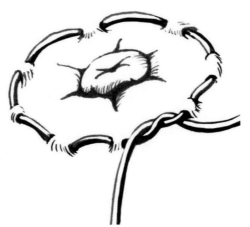

Fig. 14.20. Purse-string suture

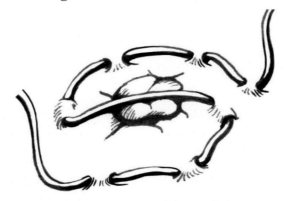

Fig. 14.21. Semi-purse-string suture

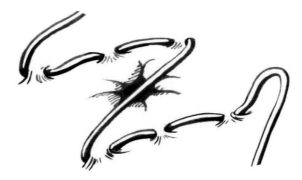

Fig. 14.22. Z-shaped suture

The steps for making a purse-string suture are shown in Figs. 14.23, 14.24.

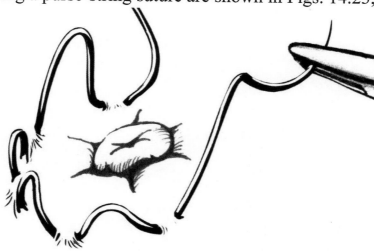

Fig. 14.23. Making a purse-string suture (stitching of tissues in a circle)

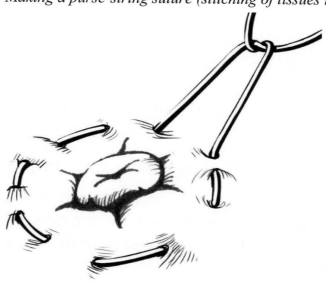

Fig. 14.24. Making a purse-string suture (tightening the first loop)

Task. Make Z-shaped, purse-string and semi-purse-string sutures on the training device (five or six stitches in a circle with diameter of 3 cm).

TEST QUESTIONS AND TASKS

14.1. What should be the ratio between the depth of tissue suturing (a), the intervals between neighbouring stitches (b) and the distances between the punctures (c) in simple interrupted skin sutures (Fig. 14.25).

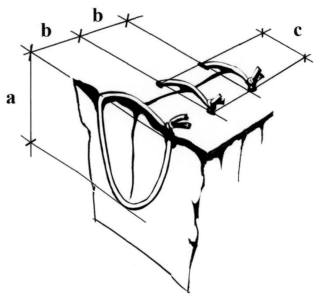

Fig. 14.25. Ratio of distances in simple interrupted skin sutures. See the description in the text

14.2. A Donati suture includes a stitch through the dermis and a stitch through the skin. Decide which is easier to start from – the dermis or the skin.

14.3. Fix drainage tubes on the training device using different sutures: with or without a bridle, passing both threads around the drainage tube and then passing only one thread. Compare how securely the tube is fixed by these different methods.

TOPIC 15.

SURGICAL SCRUBBING

Surgical scrubbing of the hands is essential before any surgical operation and is a professional duty to yourself, the patient, your colleagues and the clinic.

There are some minor variations between local rules for surgical hand scrubbing, but the basic principles are the same everywhere, including a universal standard for movement of the hands in such scrubbing (Fig. 15.1–15.6). Treatment of the front and back surfaces of the forearms up to the upper third of the arm are also fundamental (Figs. 15.7, 15.8). The use of disposable sterile brushes or sponges for hand washing is only permissible if the surgeon's skin has been heavily soiled.

All of the following standard movements for scrubbing have been established for specific and good reasons:

• The palms of the hands face each other with fingers together (Fig. 15.1);

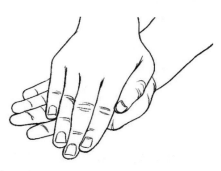

Fig. 15.1. The palms of the hands are placed against each other with fingers together

• Each hand in turn rubs the back of the other hand with fingers open (Fig. 15.2);

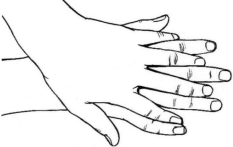

Fig. 15.2. One hand rubs the back of the other (the movement is then repeated with the roles reversed)

• The palms of the hands are placed against each other with fingers open (Fig. 15.3);

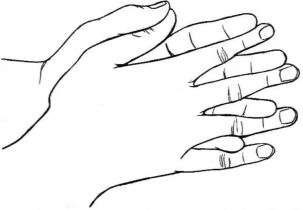

Fig. 15.3. The palms of the hands are placed against each other with fingers open

• Movements in the "lock" position (Fig. 15.4);

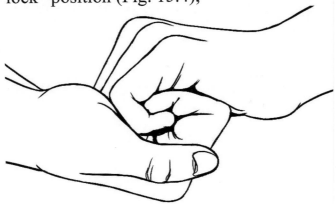

Fig. 15.4. The "lock" position

• Treatment of the thumbs (each hand in turn) (Fig. 15.5);

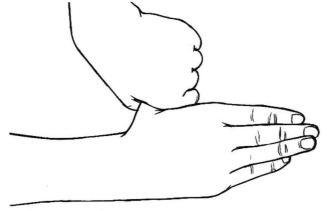

Fig. 15.5. Treatment of the thumbs (each hand in turn)

• Treatment of the palms and fingertips (each hand in turn) (Fig. 15.6, 15.7, 15.8).

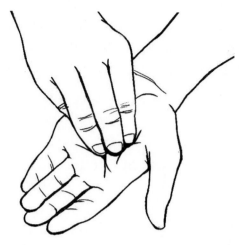

Fig. 15.6. Treatment of the palms and fingertips (each hand in turn)

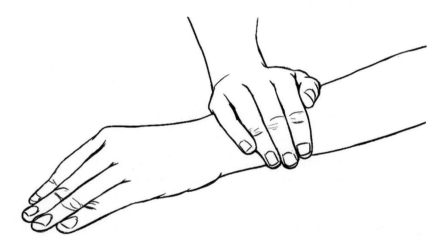

Fig. 15.7. Treatment of the front of the forearm (each arm in turn)

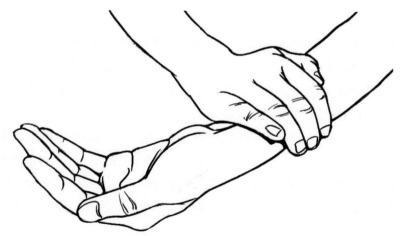

Fig. 15.8. Treatment of the back of the forearm (each arm in turn)

"In turn" means that movements are to performed alternately with the right and left hands. The sequence of movements should be strictly followed. Each movement is to be performed 10 times during one cycle. After two soapings and rinsings, the skin should be dried with a sterile cloth (first the hand and then the forearm).

Antiseptic is then applied to the skin twice, and it is rubbed in until the skin is completely dry (this sequence must be strictly observed).

Particular attention should be paid to preventing cracks and calluses on the skin, to deburring, and to keeping fingernails as short as possible, since microorganisms accumulate in great quantities under the fingernails, at the nail edges and in cracks of the skin.

When a surgeon does housework or gardening, which may involve pollution and/or injury to the skin of the hands he/she should always wear gloves. Proper hand care should be considered an essential part of preparations for work.

Task. Practise surgical hand scrubbing movements until they become automatic.

TEST QUESTIONS AND TASKS

15.1. Name the movements for surgical hand scrubbing in their correct sequence.
15.2. List the movements that apply only to surgical hand scrubbing.

CONCLUSION

Proper mastering of the studies and exercises described in this book should not be viewed as the end of a course of training, at which ultimate proficiency has been attained. Rather it should be viewed as the start of a long professional journey, in the course of which each surgeon develops the practical skills that he/she needs.

Not every skill can be learnt in advance. Often what is important for a surgeon is not whether he/she has a particular skill, but how quickly he/she can learn a new one. But the speed with which new skills can be learnt depends on how many skills have already been mastered. The more skills a surgeon already has, the easier it is to learn new ones, since many of their elements are the same.

Of course, the exercises with matches described at the start of the book will seem redundant if the surgeon has begun professional practice and the making of loops and knots has become second nature. But if these actions have not yet become absolutely fluent and automatic, it is important to maintain and consolidate proficiency. Otherwise skills are lost and bad habits are formed.

How many times and for how long the exercises are repeated, and the order in which they are carried out are for the student to decide. All of the exercises are designed to develop proficiency in the actions, which the surgeon has to carry out most often in his/her practice. After mastering all of the materials described in the book, you can repeat the tasks in any order.

ANSWERS TO TEST QUESTIONS AND TASKS

Topic 1. First exercises. Training plan. Training device

1.1. All of exercises with matches (match picking, well building, berry picking) can be carried out simultaneously with both hands.

1.2. The parts of a surgical clamp are the rings, ratchet, shank, jaws and tip.

1.3. Finger 1 has been pushed right into the upper ring, finger 5 (instead of finger 3 or 4) has been inserted into the lower ring, and the clamp is held with the concave side facing away from the midline.

1.4. This is a pressure grip with fingers 4–5.

1.5. The lace should be about 60 cm long.

1.6. The elastic tubes held in tension on the training device between two spherical holders imitate the two edges of a wound. The optimal stance of the surgeon has the wound edges parallel to a straight line between his/her elbows.

1.7. Passing the thread from hand to hand is less ergonomic, makes knot tying take longer, and can lead to various mistakes (twisting of the threads, etc.).

Topic 2. Loops and knots

2.1. A loop is made when the start and end of the thread are intertwined to make a knot.

2.2. In Fig. 2.19 the part of the knot which is circled is the first loop. This is a crossed knot +1+1.

2.3. This is a double left loop −2.

2.4. In Fig. 2.22: (a) shows a right loop and (b) shows a left loop.

2.5. The knots in Fig. 2.22 are: (a) +1−1+1−1, triple square knot; (b) +2−2+2−2, triple academic knot; (c) +2−1+1−1, triple surgical knot.

2.6. A left loop will be made. The thread grip does not matter.

2.7. Because each time a new loop is made, each tip of the thread changes its position (it is alternatively the start and end of the thread) and the hands also change their position. Direction of the hand motions in Fig. 2.23a will make a left loop and those in Fig. 2.23b will make a right loop.

2.8. The right hand is in supination and the left hand is in pronation.

Topic 3. Front and rear techniques of loop formation

3.1. Fig. 3.21 shows a pressure grip with fingers 3–5 of the right hand. It is used in both the front and rear methods of loop creation.

3.2. A left loop will be made in all cases. These thread grips (pressure grips with fingers 3–5) permit the rear method with the right hand or the front method with the left hand.

3.3. Creating the thread crossover and the loop.

3.4. Fig. 3.23 shows a simple right loop. The loop is being tightened in the correct direction, but the hands are too far away from it (this will make it hard to control tension of the threads in the loop).

3.5. The principle of alternation of techniques states that knots can be made with one hand only, alternating the methods for the end and start of the thread. This approach means that loops can be made using the same end of the thread all the time. This is valuable in practice because it makes it possible to use only one end of the thread to make loops and knots – the end that does not carry the needle.

Topic 4. Use of a clamp in the front and rear techniques of loop formation

4.1. With sufficient training, the speeds are similar. Using a clamp makes it easier to work with short and slippery threads.

4.2. Using a clamp to make knots saves thread (because a shorter thread can be used).

4.3. Finger 2 of the left hand needs to be brought close to the knot. The other thread is stretched with a clamp.

Topic 5. Making a complex loop by the front and rear techniques

5.1. The second loop is important because it is the loop that completes the knot, in conjunction with the first loop.

5.2. Friction and weaving of the threads in the first loop are what prevent it coming undone, so a complex loop is more resistant to coming undone than a simple one. Tension of the threads between the first and second loops also stop the first loop coming undone, so such tension is specially maintained while the second loop is being made and tightened.

5.3. The structure of the surgical knot includes one complex loop. The academic knot consists exclusively of complex loops.

5.4. Creation of simple and complex loops with a clamp is similar.

Topic 6. Lower and lower mirror techniques of loop creation

6.1. Use of the lower method with the right hand and lower mirror method with the left hand is possible.

6.2. Each method of loop creation can be performed with either hand. The front and lower mirror methods are for the hand holding the end of the thread, while the rear and lower methods are for the hand holding the start of the thread. So, the methods can be used in alternation.

6.3. Yes, it is possible. The end of the thread is held in the left hand by a pressure grip with fingers 1–3, so the lower mirror method is possible. After a loop has been made, the lower method can then be used for the start of the thread in the left hand.

6.4. Subjective assessments may differ, but it is definitely true that the front and rear methods are optimal for making second loops.

6.5. In the two-step technique for complex loops, the loop is made by successive operations, while in the single-step technique it is made at once. But the "speed" of the single-step method is not a significant advantage. It may be harder to execute in gloves (especially with thin, sticky threads) and it does not permit the thread to be kept in constant tension, so it is not suitable for making the second loop. The main reason for learning it is to practise synchronous hand movement and become more adept at one-step techniques.

Topic 7. Loop creation by the wind-around method

7.1. When making loops by the wind-around method with a clamp, the basic rule is followed: the loop will be on the same side as the hand (left or right), which holds the end of the thread. If the clamp in the right hand holds the end of the thread, a right loop will be created, and if the clamp holds the start of the thread, a left loop will be created. The clamp is always positioned between the start and end of the thread.

7.2. The clamp should always be positioned between the start and end of the thread, but in Fig. 7.13 it has been positioned on the outer side of the end of the thread.

7.3. This method is used only rarely in practice, if, for example, the thread ends are particularly short due to partial breakage of one or even both of them or if the threads are under strong tension in hard tissues. The technique will be necessary in such situations.

Topic 8. Various types of knot

8.1. When the lace ends are pulled in opposite directions, all of the running simple knots come undone.

8.2. The Aberdeen knot saves thread and lets you continue the suture after making the knot.

8.3. The sliding square knot easily comes undone.

8.4. In practice, use of different thread types to make a Roeder knot gives loops with different properties, and that should be borne in mind when preparing to carry out a surgical operation. You may have felt the difference when using laces made from different materials.

Topic 9. Direction of loop tightening, position of knots

9.1. This exercise will require much practice. The classic, piston-like hand movements are not possible at an angle to the training device. The direction of loop-making has to be maintained by movement of the hands and fingers. It is important to follow the rules for thread movement. Notice that it may not be possible to check correct direction of loop tightening by sight.

9.2. The knots may differ slightly, probably due to quality of the laces used or twisting of the loops when they are tightened parallel to the wound. In parallel tightening, the loops always alternate (right–left), but loop tightening always goes parallel to the wound: for the right hand, to the right; for the left hand, to the left.

9.3. Loop tightening parallel to the wound will probably feel more ergonomic in such conditions. The conditions simulated here are common in practice, so it is important to master this method. However, the loops should be tightened perpendicular to the wound, if possible.

9.4. In most cases, the knot can be shifted, but, in practice, it causes the thread to be pulled through tissue at high tension and with excessive friction, leading to damage and eruption of tissues, and the weakening of all loops in the knot. Such a shift is not recommended in practice.

Topic 10. Securing and releasing the thread with the clamp

10.1. In practice, a middle way is the most ergonomic. Use the clamp to make the thread crossover (front or rear method), and then remove the clamp and finish the loop and knot with hands only.

10.2. If two surgeons are working together in the operating theatre, they usually stand opposite each other at the operating table. Usually the main surgeon puts on the clamp, and the assistant removes it. Since the main surgeon usually puts on the clamp with the right hand, the assistant has to remove it with his/her left hand, since it is not recommended to turn a hemostatic clamp.

10.3. The clamp should be opened smoothly, without jerks, to prevent sudden movement of the vessel or tissues, which it was holding.

Topic 11. Use of scissors and scalpel

11.1. Holding the scissors this way increases the risk of injury, movements of fingers 1 and 3 are limited, transition of the scissors to a working position is complicated.

11.2. Triangular scalpels (№ 11 and № 12) are better suited for short incisions, curved (№ 10 and № 20) are better for long incisions.

11.3. Dealing with excessively long threads is easy. The best way is to grip the thread ends in a clamp, pull them taut and cut them with scissors to the right level. Leaving extra length of suture material is not recommended, except for a removable suture on the skin.

11.4. The parts of a scalpel blade are: tip, cutting edge, mounting hole, base, spine.

11.5. It is best to position both thread and scissors at an angle, as shown in Fig. 11.25b.

Topic 12. Suture material

12.1. If threads made of different materials have the same thickness, monofilament thread offers the least friction, followed by braid thread with polymer coating and plain braid thread. Twisted thread has the greatest friction (it is no longer used in surgery).

12.2. Threads made of polyglycolide and polydioxanone are absorbable.

12.3. The labels identify the following needles: a – round-piercing; b – round with cutting tip; c – reverse cutting.

12.4. Cutting needles are generally used for sutures on the skin and other dense tissues, for which a needle with large curvature is not necessary; 3/8 curvature is most commonly used.

A piercing needle with 1/2 curvature is best suited for suturing a large amount of soft tissue.

Topic 13. Using needle holder and forceps

13.1. Grip of the needle holder with fingers 1 and 4 or 1 and 3 gives firm control of the instrument, but somewhat limits freedom of hand movement. Gripping the needle holder in the palm of the hand makes it more manoeuvrable, but transition to one of the finger grips may be necessary for opening the instrument.

13.2. The position of the needle in the needle holder is optimal at 1/3 to 1/2 distance from eye, i.e. part (a) should be shorter than or equal to (b). A hold-point more distant from the eye enables stitching of denser tissue without risk of bending or breaking the needle. The needle should be gripped as close as possible to the tip of the needle holder. Observe safety precautions.

13.3. One factor to take into account is the structure of the needle itself – its curvature and length. Collect several needle types in a container for practice purposes. Observe safety precautions. Also makes sure that the needle holder and forceps are of adequate quality. The forceps should grip the needle firmly.

Topic 14. Various types of suture

14.1. You should try to ensure that the distance between neighbouring sutures (b) and the distance between punctures (c) are approximately equal, but less than the depth of suturing of the tissue (a).

14.2. The standard approach is to stitch the dermis first. The skin is then stitched by pulling the dermis up with both ends of the thread, so that (assuming the needle is long enough) both wound edges can be sewn simultaneously.

14.3. Fixing of the drainage tube with a bridle and both threads around the tube will be the most secure.

Topic 15. Surgical scrubbing

15.1. Hygiene treatment of hands consists of the following steps:
   a – the fronts of the hands are placed against each with fingers closed;
   b – each hand rubs the back of the other hand in turn;
   c – the palms of the hands are rubbed together with fingers open;
   d – lateral movement of the hands in "locked" position;
   e – treatment of the thumbs (in turn);

f – treatment of palms and fingertips (in turn).

15.2. Surgical hand scrubbing differs from ordinary hygienic treatment by the addition of two more steps:

g – treatment of the front and back of the forearms (in turn);

h – treatment of the back surface of the forearm (in turn).

REFERENCES

Boros, M. Surgical Techniques. Szeged, 2006.

Jain, S. K., Stoker, D.L., Tanwar, R. Basic Surgical Skills and Techniques. New Delhi, 2013.

Kirk, R.M. Basic Surgical Techniques (6th edition). Elsevier, 2010.

Murtagh, J. Zabiegi Lekarskie [in Polish]. Warsaw, 1995.

Ratner, G.L. Tips for a Young Surgeon [in Russian]. Samara, 1991.

Schein, M., Rogers, P.N. M. Schein's Common Sense Emergency Abdominal Surgery. Berlin, Heidelberg, New York, 2005.

Semenov, G.M. Modern Surgical Instruments [in Russian]. St. Petersburg, 2012.

Sherris, D.A., Kern, E.B. Essential Surgical Skills. Philadelphia, London, 2004.

Simbirtsev, S.A. (Ed.). Basics of Operative Surgery [in Russian]. St. Petersburg, 2002.

Sleptsov, I.V., Chernikov R.A. Knots in Surgery [in Russian]. St. Petersburg, 2000.

Whalan, C. Assisting at Surgical Operations – A Practical Guide. Cambridge, 2006.

Zubarev, P.N. (Ed.). Practice of General Surgery [in Russian]. St. Petersburg, 2004.

Printed in Great Britain
by Amazon

82590705R00112